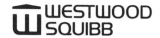

WESTWOOD SQUIBB

100 Forest Avenue Buffalo, NY 14213-1091
716 887-3400 Telex: 883988

Dear Reader:

Westwood-Squibb Pharmaceuticals and your doctor are pleased to make this book, "Managing Your Psoriasis" by Nicholas Lowe, M.D., available to you.

"Managing Your Psoriasis" provides the latest in medical thinking on psoriasis and offers practical advice on handling the disease.

Westwood-Squibb, a division of Bristol-Myers Squibb, is the nation's largest research and development facility devoted to the specialty of dermatology. Together with your doctor, we are dedicated to providing the highest quality products and services for your skin care needs.

Sincerely,

Jeff Marsh
President
Westwood-Squibb Pharmaceuticals
Buffalo, New York

MANAGING
YOUR
Nicholas J. Lowe, M.D.
PSORIASIS

MASTERMEDIA LIMITED
NEW YORK

MASTERMEDIA and colophon are registered trademarks
of MasterMedia Limited.

Library of Congress Cataloging-in-Publications Data

Lowe, Nicholas J.
    Managing your psoriasis / Nicholas J. Lowe.
        p.   cm.
    ISBN 0-942361-84-9 : $17.95.   ISBN 0-942361-83-0 (pbk.) : $10.95
    1. Psoriasis—Popular works.   I. Title.
RL.321.L675 1993
616.5'26—dc20   93-30165
                                                                    CIP

Designed by Jacqueline Schuman
Production services by Martin Cook Associates, Ltd.
Manufactured in the United States of America

10 9 8 7 6 5 4 3 2 1

Contents

Acknowledgments

I want to give special thanks to my wife, Pam, who has been a constant source of support and advice in establishing and refining the Southern California Dermatology and Psoriasis Centers. She and my daughters, Nichola and Philippa, have given me the understanding and support that have allowed me the time to complete this project.

I would also like to thank Judy Gruen for her superb assistance in the preparation of this manuscript.

I want to especially acknowledge the many lessons I have learned from my patients with psoriasis. They have to live with a capricious, unpredictable, emotionally draining, and occasionally disabling disease. They need our understanding, support, and encouragement. It is important for them to know of progress being made in the understanding and treatment of psoriasis so they may be encouraged about new options for their treatment.

Foreword

This book meets the urgent need for a nationally distributed, comprehensive, single-volume source of information on psoriasis for the public. Its complete review of the types of psoriasis and all the treatments provides the reader with an informative context by which to compare the merits of the various psoriasis treatment alternatives.

Improvements in technology and clinical research have improved the efficacy of traditional psoriasis therapies and generated new ones. We also have developed a greater understanding of what triggers psoriasis. Thousands of people with psoriasis have an improved quality of life as a result. Dr. Lowe has been in the forefront of developing these new therapies and broadening our understanding of psoriasis. As a nationally-recognized expert in treating this disorder, he has raised the standards in treating psoriasis. This book reflects his many years of experience in working with people to effectively cope with their psoriasis.

The NPF as a volunteer, nonprofit organization was established by people living with psoriasis and their families to help people affected by psoriasis regain control of their lives. Since knowledge is critical for anyone trying to successfully cope with psoriasis, the NPF places a high priority on education. Through its national membership newsletters and consumer booklets, NPF educates people about psoriasis and serves as a clearinghouse for the latest information relating to treatment and research. Dr. Lowe, as a member of the NPF's medical advisory board for eleven years, has been an important contributor to this national databank.

People living with psoriasis often find themselves on a frustrating quest for information about the disorder. This book responds to that need by providing a unique educational opportunity for the millions of Americans living with psoriasis to have easy access to information on psoriasis and the "state of the art" in psoriasis therapy.

—Gail M. Zimmerman
Executive Director
National Psoriasis Foundation

MANAGING YOUR PSORIASIS

1

Introduction

"The heartbreak of psoriasis." For at least five million Americans, this is more than an advertising slogan—it's a harsh reality of life. Psoriasis is one of the most common skin diseases, affecting one in 50 adults. And psoriasis is more than a physical malady. Its markings can make patients feel ashamed and unattractive, which can lead to psychological distress. And when the skin symptoms combine with related ailments like psoriatic arthritis, patients can understandably become depressed and disabled.

In his memoirs, in a chapter called "At War with My Skin," novelist John Updike wrote that "psoriasis has the volatility of a disease, the sense of another presence cooccupying your body and singling you out from the happy herds of healthy, normal mankind. . . ." In the past, many psoriasis sufferers had to live with the knowledge that they could suffer an outbreak of their painful and uncomfortable disease at any time—usually the least convenient time, as Murphy's law would have it. And until now, many have become understandably frustrated with

1

physicians they think can't understand the vagaries of their disease or don't care enough to find cures that really work safely.

But psoriasis treatments are changing. We in the medical community, and researchers at drug companies, are developing new treatments and improving old ones. Dermatologists have a clearer understanding than ever of how current treatments actually work. Until recently, we had proof that some of them worked, but no precise understanding of how. We also have a clearer understanding of how psoriasis develops. And once we understand its development fully, we will be able to stop the development process before the disease is full-blown—or even eliminate people's susceptibility to psoriasis altogether.

Several well-respected scientists are probing the possibility that genetic factors cause psoriasis. They haven't yet determined if a single gene is the culprit, but if it is, we'll be able to take a giant step forward. If researchers identify a single psoriasis-causing gene, they may be able to find ways to alter the gene so that it doesn't send psoriasis-causing messages to the skin. That would cure psoriasis forever. Once the stuff of horror movies and nightmares, genetic engineering is now the hook many researchers are hanging their most optimistic dreams on! Until a definitive cure is found, knowledge of the increasingly-good treatment options available can make a big difference in the daily life of a person with psoriasis.

This book is designed to provide understandable information about psoriasis, and I hope it will also serve to encourage patients who feel overwhelmed by their symptoms and their frustrations. In the following chapters, I will outline the different treatments currently available (both by prescription and over-the-counter) and discuss their benefits, drawbacks, and proper uses. There *are* effective ways to cope with psoriasis—successful ways to minimize the disease's discomforts and distresses. With appropriate medical treatment, psychological counseling, relaxation techniques, home therapy and the support of family and friends, you can reduce the impact of psoriasis, and lead a more comfortable, fulfilling life.

2

What Is Psoriasis?

No one fully understands what causes psoriasis yet, but doctors have several theories. We have known for a long time that psoriasis seems to run in families. This isn't to say that if you have the disease your children definitely will, or that if your parents didn't you won't either. Rather, there is a marked increase in psoriasis among people whose parents, grandparents or siblings have the disease. If one spouse has psoriasis, a couple's children have a one-in-four chance of developing psoriasis too. If both parents have psoriasis, there is a 50–50 chance their children will inherit the disease. If one fraternal twin has psoriasis, there's a 70 percent the other will, and there's a 90 percent chance that if one identical twin has the disease, so will the other.

Although we have nailed down the numbers, dermatologists and genetics experts still don't know exactly *how* psoriasis is passed from one generation to the next. But we are getting closer to an answer. Studying blood types called HLA types has suggested to researchers that there is a specific gene that transmits psoriasis. They believe the gene is located near chromosome 6. The exact location of the gene remains unknown (there are millions of genes on each of the 26 chromosomes), but scientists are currently trying to identify that gene precisely, so that they can start experimenting with it and alter the way it affects people who are born with it.

CORRECT DIAGNOSIS OF PSORIASIS

Proper diagnosis of your psoriasis is your best assurance of proper treatment. Many physicians who are not dermatologists see very few patients with psoriasis. Your family physician may have difficulty in pinpointing the diagnosis, which could lead to inappropriate treatment. That's why it is important to consult a dermatologist at the early stages of psoriasis.

Trained dermatologists can usually diagnose psoriasis simply by looking at the skin and other key areas where the disease can manifest itself (for example, in the nails). Dermatologists may, however, have a harder time diagnosing unusual instances of psoriasis or cases that have been incompletely treated by another physician. Under these circumstances, the doctor may have to wait for you to develop more typical features of psoriasis before confirming the diagnosis.

In some cases, your dermatologist may suggest a skin biopsy to aid in the diagnosis. This is a very simple and relatively painless procedure. In a skin biopsy, the doctor takes very small samples of the skin, which has been numbed by a local anesthetic. These skin biopsies can then be examined under the microscope and can reveal certain characteristics of psoriasis that will help the dermatologist diagnose your psoriasis and devise a treatment plan that will work for you.

If your dermatologist only treats mild cases of the disease, he or she may refer you to a psoriasis specialist who has more advanced facilities at his or her disposal.

The Role of the Dermatologist
It is important to note that dermatologists can be and should be extremely supportive and positive when dealing with psoriasis. It is also important for the psoriasis patient to realize that:

- *Many treatments are available* to control their disease.
- Their disease can *improve maximally or clear up for prolonged periods of time* with the correct use of different forms of treatment.
- In addition to the possibility of disease remission, the *impact of the disease on their daily lives can be reduced significantly.*
- Support groups, psychotherapy and counseling can lead to a *major improvement in feelings of self-esteem and ability to cope with the disease.*
- Many new effective treatments have become available over the last decade and newer treatments being researched at present will result in *improvements in treatment for many psoriasis patients over the next decade.*

The purpose of this book is to assist the psoriasis patient in dealing with their disease and to provide them with positive information about major improvements in the treatment of the disease which may result in many patients' lives being considerably improved over the next decade, as these new treatments become available.

There is no getting around the fact that psoriasis can be a difficult disease to live with. In moderate to severe cases, patients experience pain, itching and frustration at the lack of a "cure." Their self-images can plummet. They understandably become sick of the messy creams and smelly tars they may be using.

3

What Causes Psoriasis Skin to Look as it Does?

Beyond understanding how psoriasis is inherited, researchers have several theories as to how psoriasis actually develops in people with a genetic predisposition to it. One theory is that a lack of control of the outer skin cells leads to the greatly increased production of cells that characterize psoriasis. This, in turn, may lead to an abnormality of the blood vessels and the inflammation characteristic of psoriasis.

Other researchers feel that psoriasis patients have an abnormality in the skin that allows inflammation in psoriasis and that it is the inflammation that leads to a buildup of white blood cells from the blood. This buildup of white blood cells then triggers the thickened skin of psoriasis.

Still another possibility is that the epidermal skin cells fail to mature into the flat, thickened "cornified" layer they're supposed to. As a result, the epidermis tries to produce more cells than usual, leading to the thickened buildup of the epidermis as well as an inflammation. (See Figure 1.)

Figure 1

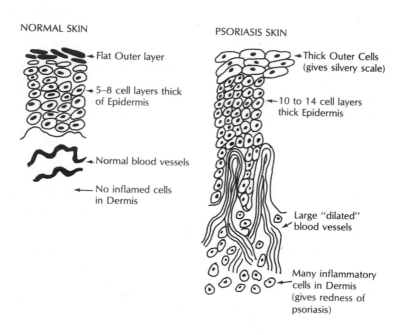

NORMAL SKIN

← Flat Outer layer

← 5–8 cell layers thick of Epidermis

← Normal blood vessels

← No inflamed cells in Dermis

PSORIASIS SKIN

← Thick Outer Cells (gives silvery scale)

← 10 to 14 cell layers thick Epidermis

Large "dilated" blood vessels

Many inflammatory cells in Dermis (gives redness of psoriasis)

Finally, a more recent theory on the causes of psoriasis has suggested that there may be an abnormal immune reaction in skin with psoriasis. The precise abnormality is not known; it may be a lack of control of certain cells in the skin that regulate the immune system. This has been suggested because of the promising results doctors have obtained with the immune-regulating drug called Cyclosporin. Researchers believe that Cyclosporin may actually correct a local change of immunity in the skin. (I will discuss Cyclosporin in more detail in Chapter 11.)

Not everyone who suffers from psoriasis suffers in the

same way, and each patient may find that symptoms vary over time. There are various reasons for this. First, infections may prompt or worsen psoriasis. For example, guttate psoriasis sometimes flares up in patients who are sensitive to bacterial (streptococcal) sore throats. Some people may get severe psoriasis on the skin fold and scalp as a result of a yeast infection in the skin. Stress has also been named as a major culprit in psoriasis flare-ups. Fortunately, counseling and relaxation techniques can go a long way to minimizing the stress-trigger and can be very helpful in keeping psoriasis under control.

It is important to know that the great majority of patients with psoriasis do not have any internal immune suppression. However, investigators who have observed people suffering from both AIDS and psoriasis have found that at some stage in the progression of AIDS, psoriasis worsens. This may also suggest that an increase or decrease in the body's immune system does indeed influence psoriasis. Researchers are pursuing this new path of study.

Let me stress that most people with psoriasis do *NOT* have immune deficiency, nor are they at increased risk of contracting AIDS. If there is an abnormal immune function in the skin, it is likely to affect only the skin. People with psoriasis do not display any evidence of general changes in their body's immunoregulatory systems.

4

Are There Different Types of Psoriasis?

Psoriasis reveals itself in many ways. The following are the most common varieties. You may well recognize them as the kind that you, a family member, or friends are coping with.

COMMON PLAQUE (PATCH) PSORIASIS

Common psoriasis, also known as psoriasis vulgaris, is by far the most common type of psoriasis, accounting for 80 to 90 percent of all psoriasis patients. Plaque psoriasis appears as raised red scaling patches. The scales, which are often silvery and thickened, appear most frequently on the elbows, knees, scalp and lower back. However, all parts of the skin may occasionally be subject to psoriasis.

GUTTATE PSORIASIS

This type of psoriasis often starts in childhood or the teen-age years, frequently with the sudden onset of small, raindrop-like patches of scaling skin, much thinner than plaque psoriasis. (It is possible for these patches to increase in thickness.) Often a sore throat of streptococcal infection will prompt the appearance of guttate psoriasis. (See the case study of Lillian in Chapter 13 as an example.)

Guttate psoriasis often covers large parts of the body. But although it can be severe, it responds very rapidly to ultraviolet therapy and other forms of treatment. It can also clear up, leaving the patient free of further outbreaks of guttate psoriasis. In such cases, localized patches or plaques of psoriasis may develop later in life.

SKIN FOLD, "FLEXURAL" AND GENITAL PSORIASIS

This type of psoriasis frequently flares up in association with more common types of psoriasis, and can cause great discomfort when one part of the skin rubs against another. This discomfort can be so severe as to become disabling for the patient. Psoriasis can occur in genital areas, which can lead to discomfort and difficulties with sexual relations.

Skin fold psoriasis is more common and troublesome in overweight patients, because their skin tends to fold and rub against itself more. But the fact that the skin fold areas are usually haired areas has led to speculation that this type of psoriasis may come from infected hair follicles. Flexural psoriasis can also occur together with scalp psoriasis for reasons that are still unclear.

ERYTHRODERMIC OR EXFOLIATIVE PSORIASIS

When psoriasis completely covers the body, it is known as erythrodermic or exfoliative psoriasis or generalized psoriasis. Because such a large area of skin is involved, patients may feel extreme discomfort. In serious cases, patients may also encounter problems controlling body temperature, particularly in very hot or very cold climates. Older people, particularly those with heart disease and heart failure, can also suffer from accelerated heart rate due to increased blood supply flowing through the severely inflamed skin.

Fortunately, generalized exfoliative erythrodermic psoriasis occurs in fewer than 10 percent of patients. Treatments like oral methotrexate, retinoids and day-care-center therapy control the condition very effectively.

PUSTULAR PSORIASIS

Localized Pustular Psoriasis

An unusual form of the disease, pustular psoriasis is often found on the palms of the hands or the soles of the feet. It can be very uncomfortable when you're walking or working with your hands. Instead of thickened scaling patches, patients often see brownish or whitish dots surrounded by inflamed red skin. Some patients with pustular psoriasis also have plaques and patches of regular psoriasis.

Standard psoriasis treatments must be modified to treat pustular psoriasis. For example, topical cortisones on the hands and feet usually have to be covered with plastic

15

gloves or plastic wrap to enable sufficient medication to penetrate the thickened skin of the palms and soles.

Generalized Pustular Psoriasis
This is a very severe form of psoriasis in which the skin is covered with non-infected pustules, which are collections of white blood cells appearing in the skin. Patients feel very ill and frequently have fever. General pustular psoriasis of this type may be caused by a number of things, including infections, medications like lithium, or the use of systemic cortisones. It may also occur as a reaction to severe sunburn.

Generalized pustular psoriasis requires urgent dermatological care. Fortunately, though, this form of the disease is rare and affects fewer than five percent of all people with psoriasis.

5

Learning to Live
with Psoriasis

As our understanding of psoriasis deepens, doctors are coming ever-closer to a cure for this once baffling disease. But until a cure is found, there are many treatments, strategies and attitudes that can make life easier and less painful for psoriasis patients.

If you have suffered from psoriasis for a while, you probably know that stress can aggravate the condition. Avoiding stress is difficult for anyone living at the end of the twentieth century, but to make matters worse, psoriasis itself can heighten stress creating a vicious cycle of flare-ups and increased tension. And once the cycle has built up momentum, it can affect your self-esteem and can even cause problems on the job and in your social life.

Luckily, there are several ways to avoid or minimize the stresses that life and psoriasis bring with them, and more stress-minimizers are being developed every day in this "New Age." Let's face it, psoriasis patients aren't the only ones today looking for a way to turn down the volume on life for a while!

There are several ways to ease the stresses psoriasis brings with it:

- Make your friends and colleagues aware of your condition, and let them know how they can help you through the tough times. If you don't ask for support, no one will know that you need it. Enlisting friends' support is helpful not only on a practical level, but also because it will make you feel less alone in your disease.
- If you find that your psoriasis worsens at certain times of the year, avoid making big time commitments for those periods. Try to reduce the number of deadlines you face and don't plan large gatherings or social events at home. It is essential, during psoriasis outbreaks that you have sufficient time to unwind and relax.
- Don't rely on drugs or alcohol to lift you out of the depression that sometimes accompanies psoriasis. For one thing, while these substances might improve your mood temporarily, they may lead to even greater depression the morning after. Also, alcohol can be dangerous when taken in combination with some of the drugs used to treat severe psoriasis.
- Start the day with pleasant thoughts and images. Imagine that your skin is going to improve and think about the positive aspects of your life. Picture yourself in a peaceful and tranquil setting, or listen to a tape of crashing waves or rainforest noises. Relaxation tapes are available at many music stores.

If you find that your psoriasis is stressing you out even with all of these exercises or that everyday stresses are making it worse your first step should be to visit your dermatologist. Dermatologists can, and should be, extremely supportive and positive when dealing with psoriasis. If yours isn't, shop around for a new specialist. And dermatologists have a lot to be positive about today. Many new treatments are available to control psoriasis and with correct use of these treatments, your psoriasis can improve maximally or clear for prolonged periods of time. Learning about these treatments may help you not only tackle the physical symptoms of your condition, but may also give you an emotional boost. Just knowing that help is on the way can be very helpful itself!

Discussing your psoriasis and its effects with a dermatologist who understands them can go a long way to relieving anxiety, but more importantly, your dermatologist can recommend the stress-relief techniques that will work best in getting your psoriasis under control. He or she may refer you to a psychotherapist for a combination of talk therapy, stress reduction exercises and biofeedback. In addition to reducing the stress that can aggravate psoriasis, psychotherapy may help you change your responses to the psoriasis itself. Working with a good psychotherapist, you'll be able to learn new behavior patterns that can enable you to cope more effectively with your emotional concerns and to control the effect psoriasis has on your social interaction, rather than letting the disease control you.

CONSIDER JOINING A SUPPORT GROUP

If you'd like to discuss the stresses that lead to and come from psoriasis outbreaks, you may want to join a support group, instead of or in addition to one-on-one psychotherapy. In a room full of other psoriasis patients, you will soon discover that you are not the only person who is afraid or embarrassed to go to the beach. You'll learn that there are others who feel awkward exposing their skin even to close friends and family. And most importantly, you'll learn that there are ways to overcome or minimize these negative feelings and pump up your self-esteem. The best support groups are usually led by a patient, physician or psychologist who can guide all the members toward a more optimistic outlook, and support groups are most supportive when they meet frequently and are limited to about ten people. Listening to a few people speak in a huge group might be marginally helpful, but group meetings are most effective when they're small enough for you to voice your feelings and concerns every time you meet and get individual feedback from the other members.

PSYCHOTHERAPY SUPPORT

As you discuss the stresses in your life with your psychotherapist or your support-group members, you may learn first-hand what dermatologists have known for a while—It often takes several weeks between the time of the stress and the worsening of the psoriasis. You may have thought there was no connection between life's little dramas and the state of your skin. But, when you come to see the cycle's pattern, it will be easier for you to break the cycle. For example, if you discover that having a fight with your parent, child, spouse or work supervisor always results in a bad psoriatic outbreak, you may have extra incentive to find a more amicable way to settle your differences. If nothing else, recognizing exactly how and when stress affects your psoriasis will help you find the relaxation techniques that help minimize the flare-ups if you employ them soon enough after the stress trigger.

Some of the techniques that may work for you include self hypnosis, meditation and yoga. Major metropolitan centers have classes in all of these disciplines, and some psoriasis centers have support groups that can train you in these stress-reduction techniques as well.

If these stress-reduction strategies are not sufficient, you may want to consult a psychiatrist. Unlike psychologists, psychiatrists are licensed to prescribe drugs, and there are many new forms of drug therapy that are designed to reduce stress and depression. However, let me stress that these drugs must be used under the continued guidance of a psychiatrist because there are sometimes side effects to be weighed against the benefits of the drug. Some of the medicines now available include Xanax, which is an anti-anxiety, anti-panic and anti-depressant drug, and Buspar, also an anti-depressant. Your physician or psychiatrist can tell you more about specific drugs and their respective pros and cons.

A good psychologist or psychiatrist will not brush your worries aside or minimize the legitimate concerns you might have about your condition. There is no getting around the fact that psoriasis can be a difficult disease to live with. In moderate to severe cases, patients experience pain, itching and frustration at the lack of a cure. Their self-image can plummet. They become understandably fed up with the messy creams and smelly tars they may be using. They may feel embarrassed or ashamed at how they look and always wear long pants and long sleeves, even during hot summer months. Some patients can be so angry, depressed or burned out by their psoriasis that they stop treatments and wish it away. If "wishing it away" were possible, I'm sure we would all see remarkable remissions! In the years I have been treating psoriasis, I've found that patients who have been most successful in dealing with psoriasis and by successful I mean in their attitudes as well as in their physical conditions share several characteristics. First, they have made peace with their psoriasis. This doesn't mean they have given up on finding treatments that work for them. On the contrary, it means they have said to themselves, "I have psoriasis. I will not be ashamed of it or limited by it, either socially or professionally. Since I cannot change it, I will accept it and continue to treat it as best I can."

This leads us to the second main characteristic: The most successful patients are *persistent* in their treatments. It can become quite discouraging for patients to live through so many new psoriatic eruptions, especially after relishing the freedom of being clear for a few weeks or months. Unfortunately, this is often the nature of psoriasis. Patients who cope the best are those who know to expect that new outbreaks may occur and are willing to try new treatments, creams, shampoos and whatever else may be required.

As you continue to read this book and to live with psoriasis remember that you may not be able to control your skin, but you can control your attitude towards it. Accepting psoriasis as a fact of life will free up your emotional energy for more productive endeavors and should alleviate some of the stress associated with psoriasis.

6

Psoriasis in Special Sites: Scalp, Nail, Skin Fold and Genitals

SCALP PSORIASIS

Scalp psoriasis, which occurs when excessive scaling occurs together with inflammation, affects at least half of all psoriasis patients. Because scales on the scalp, face and clothing can be very obvious, this ailment can be very rough on a patient's emotional and psychological well-being. Some patients even try to scrape their severe scaling off. Don't be one of them!! Scraping damages the scalp skin and worsens psoriasis.

There is good news and bad news regarding scalp psoriasis. The good news is that with so many treatment options available, most patients can be helped. The bad news is that the scalp is one of the most difficult areas to treat, and many patients do not easily tolerate the treatment agents. Thus, frequent alterations in their medication plans are needed. It is a constant challenge to clear scalp psoriasis effectively, maintain improvements and modify treatments based on patients' reactions to the toxicity of medications.

There are a few conditions that mimic the symptoms of scalp psoriasis, but they are actually different diseases. Seborrheic dermatitis or seborrheic eczema of the scalp is probably the most common condition that looks like scalp psoriasis. If your dermatologist has prescribed anthralin be sure someone in the office (usually, it's a nurse) gives you detailed how-to's, so that you can avoid unnecessary staining and irritation. Most importantly, remember to shampoo backwards, away from the face, to prevent the anthralin from dripping onto your forehead and from there into your eyes.

Imidazole lotions or creams are effective for some patients and once they have achieved maximum improvement, patients can usually reduce their applications from daily to occasional use and still effectively control their psoriasis.

Injecting cortisone directly into the lesions of scalp psoriasis can lead to long periods of improvement for some patients with tough but localized cases. PUVA (Psoralen-ultraviolet-A) therapy may help—particularly with thin-haired patients—and sunlight therapy is sometimes effective as well.

I believe shampoos are vitally important in controlling scalp psoriasis even though there have been few scientific studies on them. Therapeutic shampoos, usually available without a doctor's prescription, usually contain coal tars, wood tars, salicylic acid, sulfur, selenium and zinc parathione or they may combine several of these agents in one shampoo. I give samples of several shampoos to my patients and allow them to select one that proves most beneficial and least irritating. I have found that some patients with blond or dyed hair resist using tar shampoos because they sometimes stain the hair. Because these shampoos can be expensive, one of my patients offered the following tip to reduce the cost.

"I apply tar soap (Polytar) as the first coat. I then apply the tar shampoo such as T-Sal, T-gel or Pentrax which are highly concentrated and require smaller quantities. A bar of tar soap lasts a very long time. For me, regular cream rinse works very well, and I prefer it to the costly dermatological products."

A prescription shampoo called Nizoral, which became available in 1990, contains ketoconazole to reduce yeasts present on scalp skin, which in turn may help scalp psoriasis in some patients.

SCALP TREATMENTS

Some Preparations for Treating Scalp Psoriasis That Are Available in the United States

Steroid preparations
Aristocort Lotion
Cordran Lotion
Cyclicort Lotion
Dermasmoothe FS Lotion
Diprolene Lotion
Diprosone Lotion
Diprolene Gel
Lidex Gel
Temovate Lotion
Valisone Lotion

SCALP TREATMENTS *(Continued)*

Purified tar preparations
Aquator Gel
Baker's P and S Plus Gel
Estar Tar Gel
Fototar Tar Cream
Psorigel
T-Derm Tar Oil
T-Derm Tar and Salicylic Acid Scalp Lotion

Salicylic acid preparations
Keralyt Gel

Other preparations
P and S Liquid

The treatments I have just outlined are recommended for localized scalp psoriasis as well as for the more generalized disease. In serious cases, you may want to go to a treatment center equipped to apply thick preparations and to remove them with specialized detergents. Our treatment center in Southern California also uses a scalp debridement machine, which aggressively shampoos the hair and removes psoriasis scale like a miniature car wash for the scalp. The patient inserts his or her scalp and a high-pressure, water-jet therapeutic shampoo moves around, reducing scalp scale and making it easier for topical therapies to work.

Patients with severe and stubborn scalp psoriasis have benefitted greatly from a systemic therapy that utilizes methotrexate or etretinate (see Chapter 11 for more on these). But because methotrexate can impair liver function, it is not appropriate for patients at risk of liver disease or those who have had drinking problems. Elderly patients should also take minimal doses.

Both methotrexate and etretinate may cause alopecia (hair loss). Etretinate should also never be prescribed to fertile women. Be sure to discuss the side effects of all drugs with your physician.

In all but the most severe cases, scalp psoriasis can be improved. It may take patience and persistence to find the right formula, but the results are well worth waiting for.

NAIL PSORIASIS

Nail psoriasis affects almost half of all people with psoriasis and 80 percent of those with psoriatic arthritis. Patients complain about changes in the appearance and texture of the fingernails more often than toenails, but this may be because patients are less likely to notice or be bothered by toenail psoriasis. Some people have psoriasis on their nails but nowhere else.

In severe cases of nail psoriasis a person can actually become disabled when trying to use their hands or fingers and even mild cases can cause some disfigurement. Psoriatic nails may lose their normal, healthy look and can become yellowed or otherwise discolored. The most frequent symptom of nail psoriasis is the appearance of pits. These are shallow depressions that are usually less than one millimeter in diameter. There may be a few isolated pits on one or two nails or on all nails.

Extensive nail psoriasis can actually cause the nails to crumble easily. Other symptoms include furrows, depressions and grooving. Nails sometimes detach themselves from the nail bed. This condition is called onycholysis. This occurs almost as often as pitting. Usually, the nail detachment begins at the edge of the nail and may spread backwards under it. The area surrounding the onycholysis may have yellowed or become brownish and can have the appearance of oil spots.

If a bacterial or fungal infection emerges in psoriatic nails, you may experience more painful swelling of the skin around the nail.

Treating generalized psoriasis is usually more effective than attempting to treat the nails locally. I have found that psoriatic nails respond to internal medications methotrexate and etretinate, for example, and to PUVA phototherapy. (See Chapter 10 and 11 for more information on these treatments.)

Unfortunately, nearly every method of local nail treatments has disadvantages. Injectable cortisones sometimes work, but the injections can be uncomfortable and there are also the possibilities of relapses and skin atrophy. Patients opting for injections usually need at least one injection every month for three to four months.

High-potency topical steroids applied under the nail may also help, but this kind of therapy must be continued for several months because nails grow slowly. Furthermore, soft tissue under the nail can atrophy before any normal nail growth emerges.

Luckily, nail psoriasis can sometimes go away all by itself. My general advice for psoriasis patients with nail disease is to try to avoid damage and injury to the nails which could prompt or worsen nail psoriasis problems.

If you have nail psoriasis,
try to follow these recommendations:

- Keep nails trimmed down to where the nail is firmly attached. This avoids putting pressure on loose nails.
- Avoid activities that might injure the nails.
- Wear gloves when working with your hands.
- Try to improve the appearance of damaged nails with artificial nails, clear or colored nail varnish.
- See your dermatologist for advice if the nails or surrounding skin becomes too uncomfortable.

SKIN FOLD AND GENITAL PSORIASIS

When psoriasis affects skin sites such as under-arms, groin and genital skin, patients may become extremely uncomfortable and often suffer considerable pain and embarrassment. Fortunately, several treatment options are available. These skin areas are very prone to irritation from some topical medications and dermatologists must use extreme caution when prescribing treatments.

My recommendations for treating these delicate skin areas include using only mild cortisone creams or ointments, with none stronger than one percent hydrocortisone. These may be combined with antifungal and anti-yeast creams because these skin areas can become easily infected with yeast such as Candida and fungi.

I avoid suggesting coal tar preparations because of the possible risk of skin cancer if they are used long term in skin fold areas particularly on genital skin. Instead, I suggest patients shampoo these sites when showering. Use a shampoo containing salicylic acid or sulphur, for example Sebulex or Nizoral. This is easy to do, and helps control the psoriasis in some patients.

For more severe cases, I recommend therapy at a treatment center with very low concentrations of anthralin (0.05%) creams. Higher strength steroid antifungal creams, such as Lotrisone, can be used for short time periods, but should be avoided long term because the strong steroid may cause groin-skin thinning.

If you suffer from genital psoriasis, you may require a short course of phototherapy. Avoid excessive phototherapy treatments however, because they may cause genital skin cancer just as tanning booths might. Low strength hydrocortisone creams are milder and may be more safely used on genital skin once the psoriasis improves.

When psoriasis affects the genital skin, both the patient and his or her sexual partner may need reassurance and encouragement. If you and your spouse or partner are concerned or put off by genital psoriasis, talk to your dermatologist together.

Remember: psoriasis is not infectious and cannot be transmitted to another person by sexual contact. Using condoms may be helpful for male patients with psoriasis on their penis and women can use lubricating jelly to reduce aggravating their psoriasis during sexual intercourse.

7

Psoriatic Arthritis

Psoriatic arthritis, which affects about ten percent of all psoriasis patients, most commonly flares up in the hands and feet. It can also cause inflammation, swelling and pain of larger joints, including the knees, elbows and hips, and the spine. Like all arthritis, psoriatic arthritis causes stiffness, pain and lack of movement in affected areas.

Psoriatic arthritis can occur in adults or children. In the vast majority (84 percent) of adults who have the condition, psoriasis alone precedes the onset of arthritis, sometimes by as much as 20 years. The skin and joints become afflicted simultaneously about ten percent of the time and often nails are affected as well.

In children, arthritis precedes psoriasis in up to 52 percent of all cases, with girls contracting psoriatic arthritis nearly three times as often as boys.

We do not know why some patients with psoriasis get arthritis. Patients who develop psoriatic arthritis in their backs, a condition known as spondylitis, often have an inherited risk for back arthritis. Other types of psoriatic arthritis do not have this hereditary link. Scientists are trying to understand the link between arthritis and psoriasis more clearly. One study shows that people with severe skin psoriasis have a greater propensity towards arthritis and another study indicates that patients with pustular psoriasis were likely to develop more severe psoriatic arthritis. In fact, many psoriatics find that their arthritis is more severe than their skin disease.

There are four main types of psoriatic arthritis afflicting adults.

Asymmetric Arthritis
By far the most frequently seen form of arthritis in psoriasis, asymmetric arthritis accounts for 70 percent of all cases. Typically, two or three joints are involved, usually on the toes or fingers. This form may also give rise to the appearance of a sausage-shaped swelling of a finger or toe, called a "sausage digit." It is often associated with finger or toe nail involvement. However, asymmetric arthritis may also involve knees, elbows, wrists and ankles.

Symmetric Polyarthritis
Symmetric polyarthritis, which occurs in up to 15 percent of patients with psoriatic arthritis, is very similar to simple rheumatoid arthritis. Your doctor will determine which of the two is causing your symptoms with x-rays and blood tests. Women are far more likely to develop symmetric polyarthritis than men.

Deforming Polyarthritis
This is a severe form of the disease that emerges in about five percent of all patients. It is characterized by sausage digits and dramatic deformities of the toes.

Spondylitis with or without Sacrolitis
Afflicting up to five percent of patients, this condition can also occur simultaneously with other kinds of psoriatic arthritis. In the early stages, it is characterized by stiffness and lower back pain. Later on, patients may develop more severe loss of back mobility.

TREATMENT OF PSORIATIC ARTHRITIS

It is very important for patients with psoriatic arthritis and psoriasis to be under a rheumatologist's care for their arthritis, and separately see a dermatologist for their skin disease. Improving and controlling the skin disease often helps the arthritis as well.

Because extensive skin psoriasis can be emotionally debilitating in itself, the additional burden of arthritis can become devastating. Therefore, managing the skin, the joints *and* the psyche are critical in an overall treatment plan. A number of treatment options are now available.

Patients suffering from prolonged joint stiffness, pain, fatigue and joint swelling need rest. Sometimes activity splints are helpful, these enable patients to maintain some function in their hands. Alternately, rest splints protect the joints and help ease inflammation and other symptoms.

Nonsteroidal anti-inflammatory drugs (NSAIDs) provide relief by reducing inflammation and pain in the joints. There are several NSAIDs available, including aspirin, but none will prompt a remission of the disease, and some may have side effects.

NONSTEROIDAL ANTI-INFLAMMATORY (ARTHRITIS) DRUGS

- Indocin
- Clinoral
- Naprosyn, Anaprox
- Voltaren
- Feldene

- Meclomen
- Motrin
- Tolectin

Less commonly used:
- Azulfidine

REMITTIVE AGENTS

If over-the-counter painkillers cannot control your condition, or if the psoriatic arthritis has become severe, your doctor may prescribe drugs to try and protect the joints from further destruction.

Methotrexate, which we have discussed earlier, is frequently used to treat other cases of severe psoriasis as well as to manage psoriatic arthritis. (See Chapter 11 for more details about methotrexate.) Other treatments for psoriatic arthritis are listed as follows:

Gold
Yes, gold. This precious metal can be injected into a muscle or taken orally and may be very valuable for some patients with psoriatic arthritis. Skin rashes may flare up as a side effect, though. Your doctor will have to monitor your blood pressure and kidney function.

> *Some side effects of nonsteroidal anti-inflammatory drugs include:*
> - kidney problems
> - skin rashes
> - sun sensitivity
> - stomach pains and heartburn
> - bleeding from the upper bowel
> - worsening of psoriasis (occasionally with indomethacin)

Antimalarial Drugs

Antimalarial drugs, such as chloroquine, hydroxychloroquine, and atabrine, can be very useful for patients with psoriatic arthritis. They must be carefully administered, however, because they can aggravate skin psoriasis. Also, all of these drugs have side effects that you'll want to weigh against the severity of your arthritis pain. Chloroquine can cause eye damage, necessitating regular visits to the eye doctor. All antimalarials may cause skin rashes and may damage liver function.

Systemic Corticosteroids

Systemic corticosteroids are usually not recommended to manage psoriatic arthritis because while they may ease symptoms, these drugs do not stop the disease's progression. Furthermore, high doses are usually required to produce any significant relief and when systemic corticosteroids are stopped, the skin psoriasis may worsen, occasionally turning into generalized pustular or exfoliative psoriasis.

Joint Injections of Corticosteroids

Local steroids, however, can be very effective when injected into inflamed joints or tendons. Joint surgery may be helpful to some patients who have deforming types of arthritis, for example, on the fingers and toes, but only when the active, inflamed stages of the arthritis subside.

8

Children and Psoriasis

Psoriasis may appear as early as birth. In fact, ten to 15 percent of all psoriasis patients first encountered their skin condition before the age of ten, and 30 percent before the age of 20. Interestingly, more girls get psoriasis than boys, though the male-female ratio is about equal in adults.

Parents who have psoriasis themselves sometimes feel guilty when their children develop it and many psoriatics agonize over whether to have children at all fearing their offspring will experience the same discomfort, pain and embarrassment they have endured. But while childhood psoriasis can be uncomfortable and embarrassing, it is also usually treatable. Identifying and understanding your child's disease are the first steps to helping him or her live with it and flourish despite the discomforts and inconveniences of psoriasis.

COMMON FORMS OF CHILDHOOD PSORIASIS

Along with the usual appearance of plaques, children also develop guttate psoriasis, often preceded by an upper respiratory infection or streptococcal infection also known as strep throat. Seek a pediatrician's care for these infections while you continue to take your child to the dermatologist for treatment of any skin symptoms.

Children are also particularly prone to seborrheic psoriasis and scalp psoriasis. Some infants are troubled by psoriasis in the usual "diaper rash" zones.

Dermatologists should use caution in prescribing a treatment plan for children, since the disease may persist throughout a lifetime and will vary in severity. High-potency topical steroids should be avoided. A medium-strength steroid is the highest dosage I would recommend for children.

Anthralin can be used in older children who are capable of keeping still during its application. Even then, parents should supervise anthralin treatments and ensure the medicine has only brief contact with the skin. I prefer to see children treated with coal tar preparations because of their relative long-term safety record. Although they aren't as powerful as steroids, tars also lack harmful side effects. Avoid long-term use of coal tars for skin fold areas (such as armpits and groin). There *is* a risk of increased skin cancers.

I believe strongly that children with more severe conditions who fail to respond to these recommended topical treatments should be treated as inpatients or at a day-care center. Goeckerman therapy, (described more fully in Chapter 13), either alone or combined with anthralin, has stood the test of time and is considered relatively safe. It also offers the chance of a reasonably long period of remission.

Fortunately, *very* few children develop severe and life-threatening psoriatic conditions. In the rare instances where it does occur, great care must be taken in selecting treatment. A short course of systemic retinoids is justified only for severe, uncontrolled erythroderma or generalized pustular psoriasis. In any case, systemic retinoid therapy should not be prolonged in children. PUVA therapy may be useful in treating severe psoriasis in children, but again, only for short periods because of the risk of skin cancer.

Parents (or prospective parents) who worry about their children becoming psoriatics should remind themselves that psoriasis sometimes disappears on its own and those that do have it can have long, successful remissions. Further, the condition can be managed very well with proper therapy.

In the meantime, there are things parents can do to help support their children through their psoriatic episodes.

- Phone your child's teacher or make an appointment to discuss the child's condition. Make sure the teacher understands that psoriasis is not contagious. Find out how other children are treating your child and ask the teacher to speak to any children who may fear or not understand why your child looks different. If other kids are picking on your child, you may want to call their parents personally.
- Set a good example for your child. When others ask questions about psoriasis, discuss it matter-of-factly without any shame or embarrassment. If you accept the condition as an objective fact, so will your child.
- For younger children, add some "play time" into medication time. Play games with ointments, (connect the

dots to draw pictures, for example). Sing songs, talk about pleasant experiences the child has or is looking forward to and give your full attention to the child. Listen to his objections when he voices them and remain sympathetic but firm about applying the prescribed medications. Try to relax with your child during these application sessions.

- Explain to your child that everyone has problems or imperfections—some are visible and others aren't. Help an older child find a hero who has overcome a physical challenge and read a book about that person.
- The National Psoriasis Foundation has a 10-minute video called "Kids With Psoriasis Need Friends Too." To purchase the tape ($45) or rent it ($5 plus return postage), write to NPF, 6600 S.W. 92nd Avenue, Suite 300, Portland, OR 97223. You can also arrange to show the tape to your child's class, particularly if peer questions and teasing have been bothering your child.
- The NPF also has a pen pal network for children who would enjoy correspondence with another child with psoriasis. Write to the above address for more information.
- Try to live life as normally as possible and minimize the impact the child's psoriasis has on the family. Don't worry excessively about future episodes or how severe they will be. Take one day at a time.

9

Topical Therapy: Steroids, Tars, Lotions and Creams

There are dozens of topical agents available to help treat psoriasis. These include steroids, tars, keratolytics, anthralin and emollients or moisturizers. This chapter will tell you a little about each of these and will help you understand when the use of a particular topical agent is called for.

STEROIDS: CORTICOSTEROIDS AND CORTISONES

Steroids can be applied as ointments, creams, lotions, aerosols or tapes. Your dermatologist will decide on the type, potency and frequency of a steroid based on your particular condition.

Thick, plaque-type psoriasis on elbows, knees, palms, soles and other thickly skinned areas tend to resist steroids and require high strength topical therapy. Alternately, lesions in body folds, the groin area, eyelids and other thinly skinned areas are usually more sensitive to steroid treatment. Topical steroids can be used to complement other forms of topical therapy, such as tar and ultraviolet light, but they are not meant to replace them. Your dermatologist will select a steroid based on the location and severity of the lesion and the steroid's strength.

Be careful when using topical steroids, they are expensive and quite potent and must be applied only as directed by a physician. Many patients misuse steroids, rubbing too much of the medication into their skin. They think that if a little is good, a lot must be better. This is absolutely not true! Use your medication sparingly and apply only to the areas directed. Steroids should not come into contact with healthy skin, nor should you apply them to other psoriatic lesions that the physician is treating with a different medication or therapy.

Furthermore, topical steroids should never be used after the psoriasis has cleared because the medication can thin out the skin. Steroids should not be applied to the face or skin folds unless otherwise directed. Should any new skin irritation, bruising, ulcers or skin infections occur, stop the treatment until you have consulted your doctor.

Given their potency, it comes as no surprise that topical steroids have side effects, which increase with the use of extremely strong agents. Fortunately, most of these side effects can be handled either by discontinuing the steroid or by introducing another medication.

Side effects are also more likely where the skin being treated is inherently thin, but even thicker skin may atrophy (become very thin). This condition can sometimes be reversed once the medication has been stopped. Thinning skin is a particular problem with babies and young children because their skin is naturally thin. As a result, most dermatologists will try to avoid long-term application of strong topical steroids in young patients.

Other side effects of steroids include acne, rosacea, secondary infections of the skin and dermatitis. Glaucoma may result from the use of topical steroids close to the eye. Only the weakest steroid agents should be used near the eye and then, only for limited amounts of time.

Tips for Using Steroids

- Apply the steroid to the skin lesion in a thin film, with your fingertip. Use sparingly.
- Never use someone else's steroids.
- Steroids range from mild to very potent. Always know the potency of your medication.
- Use the steroids only on skin areas your doctor prescribed them for. Do not, for example, apply a steroid intended for the knees to the face or groin area.
- Avoid applying stronger steroids to face and skin folds.

TABLE 1:
TOPICAL CORTICOSTEROIDS CURRENTLY AVAILABLE IN THE U.S.

Group I	Group IV
Diprolene ointment 0.5%	Aristocort cream 0.1%
Diprolene gel	Benisone ointment 0.025%
Psorcon ointment	Cordran ointment 0.05%
Temovate cream	Kenalog ointment 0.1%
Temovate ointment	Synalar cream (HP) 0.2%
Temovate lotion	Synalar ointment 0.025%
Ultravate cream	Topicort LP cream 0.05%
Ultravate ointment	

TABLE 1: *(Continued)*

GROUP
II
Cyclocort ointment 0.1%
Diprosone ointment 0.05%
Florone ointment 0.05%
Halog ointment 0.05%
Lidex cream 0.1%
Lidex ointment 0.05%
Maxivate cream
Maxivate ointment
Maxiflor ointment 0.05%
Topicort cream 0.25%
Topicort ointment 0.25%
Topsyn gel 0.05%

Group III
Aristocort cream (111) 0.5%
Diprosome cream 0.05%
Florone cream 0.05%
Maxiflor cream 0.05%
Valisone ointment 0.1%

GROUP
V
Benisone cream 0.025%
Cordran cream 0.05%
Diprosone lotion 0.02%
Kenalog cream 0.1%
Locoid cream 0.1%
Synalar cream 0.025%
Valisone cream 0.1%
Valisone lotion 0.1%
Westcort cream 0.2%
Westcort ointment

Group VI
Tridesilon cream 0.05%
Locorten cream 0.03%
Synalar solution 0.01%
Hytone 2.5%
Dexamethasone
Elocon

Group VII
Hytone 1 %
Dexamethasone
Elocon

Groups are arranged in descending order of potency. There is no significant difference of agents within any given group: within each group the compounds are arranged alphabetically, i.e. Group I are the strongest corticosteroids, Group VII the weakest.

TARS

Although there are three different types of tars used to treat skin disorders (shale, wood and coal), coal tars seem to be the most effective in controlling psoriasis. Used alone, coal tars are not very effective. But when used in conjunction with ultraviolet therapy, topical corticosteroids and/or with anthralin spray, they have proven beneficial to combat psoriasis. These combinations of tars and other therapies may be used either on an outpatient or inpatient basis.

One possible treatment plan would call for a patient with localized psoriasis to apply a topical steroid cream or ointment once or twice a day and then apply a tar preparation at night before going to bed. Your doctor will develop a regime that is appropriate for your condition and your schedule.

One annoying problem with tar is its messiness. It can stain both clothing and furnishings, so I recommend applying the tar at least 15 minutes before dressing or going to bed so that the maximum amount of tar will have been absorbed into the skin. Still, it is advisable to wear older clothing or clothing that is already stained when tar has been applied. Many purified tar gels, lotions, creams or oils are less likely to stain clothing after they have been on the skin for several minutes.

Unless your doctor advises you otherwise, avoid exposing coal tar-treated areas of the skin to the sun. Tar treatment increases the risk of sunburn. Of course, if skin infection, redness or stinging of the skin result from using tar preparations, you should suspend your treatment and consult your dermatologist. Table 2 lists some nonprescription coal tar products.

TABLE 2: TAR PRODUCTS

Aquatar Gel
Baker's P and S Plus Gel
Estar Tar Gel
Fototar Tar Cream
T-Derm Tar Oil
T-Derm Tar and Salicylic Acid Scalp Lotion

Also available as an alternative to crude coal tar:
Liquor carbonis detergents, usually between 5 percent to 20 percent concentrations in cream, ointment or oil

- Many of these products can be messy and stain your clothing and furnishings.
- Apply *small amounts* and rub them well into the skin. Use old or stained garments as clothing after applying the coal tars.
- Many purified tar gels, lotions, creams or oils will cease staining your clothes after they have been on the skin for several minutes.
- Avoid any sun exposure of coal tar-treated skin unless advised by your physician. He may advise sun or ultraviolet treatments after you apply the coal tar, but these have to be done with his advice to avoid sun burning.

Also available as additives for bathwater:
Balnetar
Doak oil

KERATOLYTICS

These clear, nongreasy lotions, creams or gels help remove very thick scales and work well in conjunction with other topical treatments, such as tar and/or Anthralin.

I usually advise patients to apply a keratolytic agent such

as salicylic acid, lactic acid or ammonium lactate lotion twice a day. Patients who combine this with their tar preparation by mixing the two together in the palm of their hand often see greater results than if they use each agent singly.

ANTHRALIN

Anthralin is a synthetic substance made from anthracene, a coal tar derivative. It has been used in the treatment of psoriasis since the 19th century.

Anthralin is a relatively safe prescription medication that can be applied as an ointment, paste, cream or stick preparation. It is less expensive, easier and safer than PUVA, methotrexate and topical steroids, and brings dramatic relief to many patients. Anthralin takes longer to work than steroids, in many cases up to six weeks. Anthralin also can irritate the skin and some patients cannot tolerate it even in small concentrations.

Anthralin has another major drawback. It is sure to stain anything it touches, including normal skin, clothing, tile grout and linoleum. Ceramic shower tiles should rinse clean, if they do not, use a little bleach. Skin staining is actually a sign that the Anthralin is working. Since it doesn't stain psoriatic skin, the staining means the skin is clearing up. The skin immediately surrounding the plaque will probably stain, but this should clear up a few weeks after the psoriasis itself has cleared. Stained skin can also be treated with salicylic acid or another keratolytic agent.

Many patients use Anthralin in conjunction with topical steroids, PUVA, systemic retinoids and tar-based therapy. Some patients can use Anthralin at home along with "Min-

49

utes" therapy. In this procedure, Anthralin cream or ointment is incorporated into an oil-in-water emulsion (Nivea oil or Eucerin, for example). The Anthralin must be fresh to be effective. Fresh Anthralin has a bright yellow color. The name of this treatment, "Minutes," is accurate: Once applied, you wash it off between 15 and 60 minutes later with liquid soap and water and an old washcloth. Then lather with a mild soap and finish with a moisturizer.

Anthralin is applied only to the psoriatic lesions and must be rubbed in well. Any excess should be wiped off. Wear plastic disposable gloves or wash your hands carefully after applying the Anthralin. The Anthralin is left in place for increasing periods of time as follows:

> Day 1—15 Minutes (If no irritation occurs)
> Day 2—30 Minutes (If no irritation occurs)
> Day 3—45 Minutes (If no irritation occurs)

After day 4, if no irritation occurs, increase to 60 minutes until clearing occurs and the lesion cannot be felt. **Do not apply Anthralin to your face or groin.** Ask your dermatologist how to treat lesions in those areas. At the end of the contact time, the Anthralin should be thoroughly washed off with soap under running water in the shower.

The following precautions will help reduce or prevent irritation.

- Do not apply Anthralin to normal skin. Normal skin becomes irritated much faster than psoriatic lesions.
- Cover all Anthralin treated areas with loose, old clothes while the Anthralin is in place. This will prevent the Anthralin on a lesion on one part of the body from rubbing

onto normal skin on another part of the body; for example, one leg onto the other leg.

- Wash hands carefully after the application and be careful not to touch an Anthralin treated area and then an untreated area.
- Keep the Anthralin away from eyes. If eye irritation occurs, rinse your eyes thoroughly and call your physician. If children are present while you are using the Anthralin, extreme caution must be taken to prevent their accidental contact with the Anthralin.

Your doctor will want to discuss your progress with this treatment at least every week or two to guide you on changing the frequency or concentration of the Anthralin treatments.

Scientists are working on improved Anthralin drugs that may produce less irritancy and staining. Another way of reducing Anthralin staining and skin irritation is by using a lotion containing tricthanolamine. This can be applied after the Anthralin has been washed off following contact of the Anthralin on the skin. This lotion reduces the amount of skin irritancy and staining produced by the Anthralin and may make it easier for the psoriasis patient to use Anthralin. In the U.S., there are two types of prescription Anthralin, Drithocream and Anthraderm. In other countries, numerous forms of Anthralins are available including a stick Anthralin.

EMOLLIENTS

Particularly valuable in helping patients with dry skin, emollients commonly used in cream or lotion form are a useful component of psoriasis therapy. Emollients seem to slow the loss of water through the skin layers that result from frequent bathing and phototherapy and also enhance the effectiveness of phototherapy. Often, patients are asked to apply an emollient immediately before phototherapy sessions.

The thicker the cream or lotion, the more effective the emollient is likely to be. Vaseline Pure Petroleum Jelly, for example, is highly effective. It is very important to use emollients after bathing or showering. Most patients are advised to apply moisturizers twice daily and to choose the one they like best to ensure that they are regularly used in order to derive the greatest benefit. You may want to use one that is light for daytime and a heavier, thicker emollient for nighttime, when the greasy nature of the emollient won't interfere with your clothing and activities. Scrupulous attention to moisturizing can relieve you of the pain of dry skin and also reduce scaling and inflammation. In addition, moisturizers have no side effects to worry about.

There are dozens of moisturizers available in any drug store, including such well known products as Lubriderm Cream or Moisture Cream or Lotion, Vaseline Dermatology Formula Cream or Lotion, Aquaphor Cream, Eucerin Cream or Lotion, Lac-Hydrin Moisture Lotion, Cetaphil, or Neutrogena Body Oil or Lotion.

TABLE 3:
MOISTURIZERS

- Acid Mantle Creme & Lotion
- Alpha Keri Shower and Bath Oil
- Aquaphor Cream
- Carmol 10 Lotion or Carmol 20 Cream
- Complex 15 Moisturizing Cream & Lotion
- Eucerin Cream (or Lotion)
- Lac-Hydrin 5% lotion
- Lac-Hydrin 12% lotion

- Lubriderm Cream (or Lotion
- Lubriderm Lubath Bath Shower Oil

- Moisturel Cream
- Moisturel Lotion
- Neutrogena Norwegian Formula Hand Cream
- Neutrogena Facial Moisturizer
- Neutrogena Body Oil
- Neutrogena Lotion for Hand and Body
- Petrolatum White U.S.P.
- Purpose Dry Skin Cream
- Shepherd's Cream Lotion, Skin Cream or Soap
- Vaseline Dermatology Formula Cream or Lotion
- Vaseline Pure Petroleum Jelly Skin Protectant

NEWER TOPICAL TREATMENTS FOR THE FUTURE

There are several new exciting topical treatments that are being studied. One of these, which is a Vitamin D3 Analogue, calcipotriol or Calcipotriene ointment, is already available in different European countries. This is an exciting new development that has shown improvement in approximately 70 percent of patients in clinical trials. Some patients achieve complete clearance with this ointment and, unlike topical corticosteroids, it does not cause skin thinning or the sudden worsening of psoriasis that sometimes follows the discontinuation of the topical corti-

53

costeroid. Calcipotriol ointment became available in some European countries in 1991, and clinical trials are in an advanced stage in the U.S.

Calcitriol, another Vitamin D ointment, also improves psoriasis, but it also seems to increase calcium levels in the blood.

NEWER ANTI-INFLAMMATION DRUGS

There are other anti-inflammation drugs, currently under investigation, that appear to control or improve the disease. Some of these drugs, derived from some of the anti-arthritis medications taken orally, may become available for the treatment of psoriasis in the next decade.

OTHER TREATMENTS

Other treatments such as new local injections of the drug fluorouracil, which slows down the rate at which psoriasis cells are produced, may become available in the next several years. Research has shown this to be a very effective treatment for localized forms of psoriasis.

Figure 2

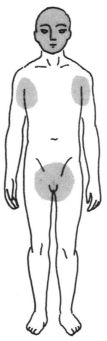

Skin areas that need extra care with topical therapies for psoriasis are shaded. Do not apply strong topical steroids, coal tars, Anthralin (dithranol), or calcipotriol (Calcipotriene Vitamin D3 analogue ointments).

10

Sunbathing, Ultraviolet and PUVA Therapy

The sun's ultraviolet rays are the most natural psoriasis treatment available. In fact, nearly 80 percent of people with psoriasis have observed that their condition improves in sunny climates. Conversely, your psoriasis may worsen in the winter, due to a lack of sunlight. Also your mood may change when the days get shorter. Hormonal or biochemical changes that occur in the winter months may also explain exacerbated winter psoriasis, but more research is still needed to confirm this theory.

Before you begin a sun treatment program, your dermatologist should take a careful history to learn how your skin reacts to sunlight exposure, and determine whether you have any existing skin cancers or have a family history of skin cancer.

People who have had skin cancer in addition to psoriasis must realize that they are at greater risk for developing new skin cancers in any part of the body and should exercise great caution when exposing themselves to the sun's powerful rays. Any areas of the skin that do not have psoriasis, such as the face, should be carefully and consistently protected with sunscreen to avoid any excessive sunlight damage and to reduce the risks of skin cancer and premature aging. Skin cancer patients undergoing sun or ultraviolet therapy should also be examined for new growths at least every four to six months.

UVB PHOTOTHERAPY

Phototherapy is often used for various skin problems including psoriasis, lichen planus, itching, eczema, mycosis fungoides, and some kinds of acne. Treatment involves exposing a patient to artificially-generated ultraviolet light for varying lengths of time. UVB phototherapy will not cure your psoriasis, but it can effectively control or improve the disease.

Typically, UVB treatments start with only a few seconds of light exposure and then gradually increase. Clearing or improvement takes an average of 15 to 20 treatments, after which your skin may stay relatively clear with one treatment every one to two weeks. Many patients may then stop treatments. Of course, each patient will vary in the number of treatments per week and the time it will take to reach clearing, but the "average" patient initially requires three to four treatments each week to clear.

Some patients may develop a mild sunburn from the UVB. If this occurs, consult your dermatologist or treatment center staff. You will not necessarily need to stop the treatment if a sunburn occurs. UVB has several other potential side effects. Patients often develop a moderate to deep suntan which usually fades within six to eight weeks after cessation of therapy. Fortunately, few Americans complain about this; despite all the dermatologists' warnings, we are still a tan-worshipping society. If you do tan from UVB therapy, you can take comfort in knowing that you're one of the few people who achieved a tan while doing something good for your body.

Unfortunately, increased incidence of skin cancer may occur later in some patients who have had many UVB treatments. Because genital skin is particularly susceptible to cancer, patients must protect the groin area during UVB therapy. And, because the light rays can also damage your eyes, you will be required to wear protective eye goggles during your light treatment.

Ultraviolet therapy is best practiced in a dermatologist's office, but this is sometimes not practical or convenient for patients who live or work too far away. If going to the doctor the three to five times a week recommended for three to six weeks is inconvenient for you, home ultraviolet therapy may be appropriate. However, many home ultraviolet machines are not powerful enough to clear patients with extensive psoriasis. Patients with more severe cases really need to be treated initially in a professional treatment center, and then they may control the disease with their home-based unit.

Before beginning this treatment, your dermatologist will want to feel relatively certain that you will improve with this regimen. You need to be instructed carefully in how to administer home ultraviolet treatments, and must remember that you need full skin examinations at a minimum of every three months while conducting home ul-traviolet therapy. Even after stopping therapy, you will require annual skin evaluations to ensure there are no signs of early skin cancer.

There are several styles of home ultraviolet therapy units which vary greatly in intensity of ultraviolet energy pro-duced. Your doctor will give you specific treatment lengths and times. Install your unit carefully. A wall-mounted tube unit should be mounted vertically at a fixed location on the wall. A line should be drawn at a set distance in front of the machine, so that you maintain a consistent level of exposure during each treatment. Follow your dermatologist's instructions carefully to avoid ultra-violet burning, and gradually increase exposure times.

When administering UVB treatments at home, you must take the following precautions:

- Wear UV protective eye glasses during treatment.
- Carefully set the machine timer as recommended by the manufacturer to avoid burning reactions.
- Visit your dermatologist every three months for routine skin examinations. This is to ensure the UV is not causing damage to your skin and that you have not developed any skin cancers. If you cannot see a dermatologist at these times, stop using the UV treatment. The impor-tance of frequent checkups cannot be emphasized strongly enough.

PUVA PHOTOTHERAPY

The photosensitizing drug known as psoralens has been used successfully with long wavelength ultraviolet light for the treatment of psoriasis in several countries. Several thousand patients have used this treatment program with good to excellent results. The psoralen capsules make the skin sensitive and responsive to the light. Without the psoralen, the light does not treat your skin condition effectively.

These drugs were first reported as being effective in the therapy of psoriasis in the early 1970s. One of the first reports of the use of PUVA using oral 8-methoxypsoralen in the treatment of psoriasis was published in 1974. Subsequently, a long-term follow-up study has confirmed the efficacy of PUVA, but certain questions regarding long-term toxicity remain. The potential problems of long-term toxicity include an increased risk of skin cancer.

Most available PUVA ultraviolet sources contain broad-spectrum UVA fluorescent bulbs. For practical purposes, these are the only light sources appropriate for PUVA phototherapy. The higher the intensity of UVA source, the shorter the treatment times required. Many different types of UVA units are available, among them upright cabinets containing 56 or more separate fluorescent tubes. Most units are vertical, but horizontal "lie-down" units are also available, and are useful for some elderly patients or patients who develop fainting episodes after long periods of standing.

PUVA phototherapy units produce significant heat, so it is important that adequate ventilation be available and air conditioning be provided in the area of the phototherapy machine. You are likely to perspire heavily during PUVA treatments, so look for a center where showers are available after your treatment.

WHO IS A GOOD PUVA CANDIDATE?

Doctors select patients for PUVA phototherapy very carefully because of the treatments' potential for long-term cumulative skin damage. PUVA phototherapy is only appropriate for those with incapacitating psoriasis, previous failure of conventional topical therapy or of tar and ultraviolet phototherapy, and rapid relapse after above forms of therapy.

Your doctor will also want to make sure that you don't have any conditions in which PUVA is contraindicated, such as photosensitive diseases, use of photosensitive drugs, previous or present skin cancers, previous x-ray therapy to the skin, or cataracts.

While oral psoralens have not been proven to produce any problem of internal disease or hepatoxicity, I still take a complete blood count and a full biochemistry panel to include liver function tests.

Before you begin your PUVA program, and later six months into the therapy, you will have to undergo an ophthalmological exam to ensure that there are no eye conditions that would preclude your taking part in the phototreatment programs. Even with an A-plus eye exam, you will have to use special plastic grey or green sunglasses on the day of the treatment program and during the light therapy.

Because some of the psoralen stays in the skin for approximately eight hours after it has been taken, it is important to avoid sun exposure after the treatment. Wear long-sleeved shirts and long pants and use plenty of sunscreen on unprotected areas. Your eyes will be more sensitive to the light during the treatment. For eight hours after you have taken the medication, wear green or grey plastic UV absorbing sunglasses outdoors.

PUVA has other potential side effects. Twenty percent of all PUVA patients experience occasional nausea and stomach upset. This can often be alleviated by taking pills with food or milk.

Psoralen capsules have not been proven safe during pregnancy, so women are advised to be using effective methods of birth control while taking part in this PUVA program.

At my treatment centers, the Southern California Dermatology and Psoriasis Centers in Santa Monica and Westlake, California, we also offer baths containing a psoralen drug. The patient bathes and then immediately receives UVA. This is very useful for patients where the psoralen pills cause nausea and sickness.

THE DEAD SEA AND SOAP LAKE: TWO NATURAL HEALING ENVIRONMENTS

The Dead Sea in Israel is the lowest point on the earth's surface, 1,312 feet below sea level. King Herod used to travel to the Dead Sea thousands of years ago to revitalize his spirit and body. Since then, thousands of people have found this region wonderfully therapeutic, particularly for psoriasis, arthritis, and eczema.

What's so special about the Dead Sea? For one thing, the additional layers of the earth's atmosphere there filter out the shorter, more harmful ultraviolet rays while allowing the longer UVA rays to penetrate. As a result, patients can expose their skin to the sun for a long time without burning. The local air is also the richest in oxygen—10 percent more than at the Mediterranean Sea level. This combination seems to produce an increased metabolic activity rate in the body while at the same time making people feel relaxed. The air near the Dead Sea also contains a high concentration of bromide, a chemical found in many sedatives.

Some physicians guess that the hydration of the skin by the Dead Sea water, which contains a disproportionately high mineral content, may also explain the area's therapeutic quality.

Patients usually remain at the Dead Sea for four to five weeks to obtain maximum improvement. Your psoriasis may reappear after you have been home for a while, but ultraviolet therapy, either in the dermatologist's office or at home, may stem the reemergence of the condition.

Your travel agent should be able to provide more details on specific Dead Sea treatment centers and the best times of year to take advantage of them. Several health insurance companies reimburse the cost of this therapy.

Those unable to travel to Israel may want to visit the small town of Soap Lake in Central Washington, a popular haven for psoriatics and arthritics. Like the Dead Sea, Soap Lake contains an unusually high mineral content located in a dry desert climate. Lake water is piped in to many of the town's motels, and hot mineral baths are also available. Reasonably priced accommodations are available during June, July and August. For more information, write to the Soap Lake Chamber of Commerce, P.O. Box 433, Soap Lake, WA 98851 or call (509)246-1821.

SUNLIGHT THERAPY

The cardinal rule of sunlight therapy for *everyone* is: Thou Shalt Not Get a Sunburn. I recommend limiting sun exposure to 15–30 minutes on each side of the body each day to start, and gradually increasing your exposure by 15 minutes every second or third day to a maximum of no more than two hours. Remember that sunburn does not show itself until the evening or even the next day, so time your sun exposure carefully. In southern parts of the country, 2 P.M. is probably the ideal time of day to begin in the summer, 12 noon in the winter. People living in the northern-most latitudes should probably begin their treatments at noon.

It may take as long as four weeks before the sun improves your psoriasis. Patients often stop sunbathing because their first few treatments seemed to make the psoriasis worse. If this happens to you, you probably allowed yourself too much sun, too fast, and inflamed your psoriasis.

Once your psoriasis has improved, you and your dermatologist should talk about the next step. In some cases, it is advisable to reduce the sunbathing to once a week, and in others, it is best to stop sunbathing altogether.

11

Oral and Injectable Medications

If you have extremely severe or disabling psoriasis, or have the disease in disfiguring parts of the body such as hands, nails, scalp and face, your physician may prescribe oral medications or intramuscular injections. You may hear your dermatologist refer to these as "systemic" medications or treatments. Since these treatments are taken internally, a dermatologist must be extremely careful in prescribing them because all have potential side effects. Make sure you are fully informed about the possible side effects of these treatments. Then judge for yourself, in consultation with your dermatologist, whether you are willing to hazard these risks in the hope that the drugs will substantially clear your condition.

There is a wide variety of oral medications, including etretinate (called Tegison in the U.S.), Isotretinoin (called Accutane in the U.S.), methotrexate, Cyclosporine, azulfidine, hydroxyurea, and Aziathioprine.

ETRETINATE OR ISOTRETINOIN

These drugs are frequently referred to as vitamin A derivatives and are also known as retinoids. Because retinoids are related to vitamin A, you should avoid taking vitamin A supplements because they may add to the unwanted side effects of Tegison. Check with your doctor or pharmacist if you have any questions about vitamin supplements.

Over the past decade, etretinate (known as Tegison in the U.S.) and Isotretinoin (called Acutane in the U.S.) have become available and have proven to be particularly successful in treating general pustular psoriasis. Patients frequently clear more completely when they have taken retinoids in conjunction with their PUVA or ultraviolet therapy than when they undergo light therapy alone. That's because the retinoid reduces the amount of ultraviolet rays needed for therapy, and the combination improves the efficacy of the treatment as a whole.

The dosage of Tegison varies from patient to patient, with the number of capsules you must take determined specifically for you by your doctor. Periodically during treatment your doctor may change the amount of medicine you need to take. Make sure you follow the schedule you are given. If you miss a dose, do not double the next dose. If you have any questions, call your doctor. You should take Tegison with food.

A dermatologist should alert you to the following possible side effects of Tegison, which include dryness of the skin, mouth and lips; hair loss; increased fat levels in the blood; altered liver function; and bony overgrowths on the skeleton (this occurs only after prolonged use of the retinoid). Furthermore, Tegison cannot be prescribed for women of child-bearing years because the drug lingers in the body long after it has been ingested and may harm a developing fetus. Fertile women can use Isotretinoin, known commercially as Accutane. It is popularly used for severe acne and is occasionally used in treating generalized pustular psoriasis. Women should avoid becoming pregnant while taking Accutane.

Tegison generally results in improvement in most patients. Some patients, in fact, have obtained complete clearing of their disease after four to nine months of therapy. You should keep in mind, however, that because some degree of relapse commonly occurs within a few months after therapy is discontinued, most patients require long-term therapy with Tegison. Also, because each patient's dosage regimen may vary, you should discuss your exact course of therapy with your doctor.

Like many patients, you may find that your psoriasis will get worse during the first month of treatment with Tegison. Occasionally patients experience more redness or itching at first, but these symptoms usually subside as treatment continues. Blood tests will be necessary before and during treatment to check your body's response to Tegison.

You may have to wait two or three months before you realize the full benefit of Tegison. In the first few weeks, perhaps before you see any healing, you may begin to have some side effects. You can expect, most often, to find peeling of the fingertips, palms and soles; chapped lips, dry skin and nose; loss of hair, eye irritation, itching, excessive thirst; bone/joint pain; rash, fatigue, red scaly face; sore mouth and skin fragility. If you develop any of these side effects, check with your doctor to determine if any change in the amount of your medication is needed. Also, ask your doctor to recommend an emollient if drying or chapping develops. If you wear contact lenses, you may find that you are less able to tolerate them during and after therapy.

Patients taking Tegison occasionally lose some hair. The extent of hair loss that you may experience and whether or not your hair will return after treatment cannot be determined.

Patients also sometimes experience decreased night vision. Since the onset of this problem can be sudden, you should be particularly careful when driving any vehicle at night. If you experience any visual difficulties, stop taking Tegison and consult your doctor.

You should be aware that Tegison may cause other serious side effects. Be alert for any of the following:

- Headaches, nausea, vomiting, blurred vision
- Changes in mood
- Persistent feeling of dryness of the eyes
- Aches or pains in bones or joints, or difficulty in moving

If you experience any of these symptoms or any other unusual or severe problems, discontinue taking Tegison and immediately check with your doctor. These problems may be the early signs of more serious side effects which, if left untreated, could result in permanent effects. Bone changes have been detected by x-ray in patients receiving Tegison. The significance of these changes is not presently known.

Your doctor generally will stop your treatment when your skin has sufficiently cleared. You may experience some degree of relapse within a few months after you stop your therapy. This is common. If you notice a *worsening* of your condition, contact your doctor. Subsequent courses of treatment will generally produce the same response as the first course.

The FDA is now considering approval of a new drug called acetretin, which accomplishes all that etretinate does except that it clears more rapidly from the body.

METHOTREXATE

Methotrexate, which has been used for psoriasis treatment longer than any other internal medication, is usually taken once a week either orally or by injection. While very effective, this drug must be used with caution and there are several limitations.

Patients must have no history of liver disease or of excessive alcohol consumption. Kidney function must also be normal so that the drug can clear itself easily from the body. Aspirin and arthritis medications could increase the toxicity of methotrexate, so consult your dermatologist before taking them. Ideally, patients should see their physicians every four weeks while on methotrexate. If the treatment lasts beyond three months, it is important to have a liver biopsy because methotrexate can cause fibrosis damage to the liver. A liver biopsy is done with a tiny needle inserted through the skin into the liver to extract a small liver sample. The procedure is done under local anesthesia.

Most side effects can be detected before they become serious, and your physician will keep you under close supervision, arranging regular visits and laboratory tests. For the safe treatment of your psoriasis, it is important that you carry out your physician's instructions faithfully and promptly report any side effects or symptoms you may develop.

HOW TO TAKE METHOTREXATE

Unlike most medications, methotrexate is given weekly, rather than daily, with the weekly dose taken either as a single or divided dose. The importance of this weekly schedule cannot be overestimated. Taking methotrexate more often or changing the dose schedule in any way can result in serious side effects. If you accidentally take your dose too often, notify your physician at once. If an accidental overdose occurs, an antidote may be necessary and must be given as early as possible.

The most common side effects of methotrexate are loss of appetite, nausea (but rarely vomiting), diarrhea, abnormal liver test results, periodic blood tests will check for this, or sores or ulcers in the mouth. If these or other problems trouble you, or if you should develop any signs of infection or unusual bleeding, notify your doctor promptly and before your next dose of methotrexate is due. These side effects are usually temporary, but changes in dose are frequently required.

Other medicines you are taking may result in an increase in side effects or a decrease in the effectiveness of methotrexate. Tell your physician about all the medicines you are taking, whether they are prescription or nonprescription medicines. Do not begin or change the dosage of any medicine without first checking with your physician. This is *especially* true of aspirin, aspirin-like drugs (the so-called nonsteroidal anti-inflammatory drugs), and antibiotics that contain the drug trimethoprim.

Unrelated medical conditions, especially dehydration, can also increase the risk of methotrexate toxicity. Abdominal upset, when accompanied by significant vomiting, diarrhea, or decreased fluid intake, can lead to dehydration. Notify your physician if these symptoms develop.

Alcoholic beverages (including beer and wine) may increase some of the side effects, including the chance of liver damage, and should be severely restricted or avoided altogether.

Side effects can occur at any time during your treatment. Periodic laboratory tests and sometimes other types of tests arranged by your physician are necessary for the safe use of methotrexate. Your cooperation is essential.

Methotrexate is known to cause birth defects and may cause miscarriage or stillbirth, especially in the first three months of pregnancy. Pregnant women must not take methotrexate, and women of childbearing age must not become pregnant while taking methotrexate. Adequate contraceptive measures are necessary during therapy and for several months thereafter. Consult your physician before considering pregnancy.

Long-term therapy may result in scarring (fibrosis or cirrhosis) in the liver. At times it may be necessary to have a liver biopsy to determine whether scarring is present. Whether and when to do a liver biopsy is a matter of discussion between you and your physician.

In addition, very rarely in psoriasis patients, methotrexate can cause a lung reaction similar to pneumonia. The symptoms are usually fever, cough (often dry and hacking), and shortness of breath (which can become severe). Notify your physician promptly should you develop such symptoms.

In summary, here are guidelines for taking methotrexate:

- Take your methotrexate weekly, not daily, in one, two, or three doses as directed by your doctor.
- Notify your physician at once if an accidental overdose is suspected.
- Notify your physician at once if you develop fever, cough, and shortness of breath.
- If any side effects develop or any symptoms of dehydration occur, notify your physician before the next dose of methotrexate.
- Do not begin or change any medicines without first checking with your physician.
- Avoid alcoholic beverages.
- Obtain the tests ordered by your physician.
- Avoid pregnancy during and for a time after methotrexate.

Despite all the precautions necessary, methotrexate remains the treatment of choice for numerous patients. It is an extremely valuable and effective drug, and there are many patients who tolerate it with no side effects at all.

CYCLOSPORINE

Initially used as an immune suppressive drug in organ transplant patients, Cyclosporine has been found to work very well and very rapidly in treating severe psoriasis. As with methotrexate, it is best not to use Cyclosporine over prolonged periods of time because the drug suppresses the body's immune system. Protracted use theoretically may lead to increased risks of cancer particularly lymphoma, although a higher cancer risk has not been seen yet in psoriasis patients treated with Cyclosporine.

As a further precaution, Cyclosporine should be taken only by patients with normal blood pressure and kidney function. Given the powerful nature of the drug, only a dermatologist experienced in its use should prescribe it.

Typically, Cyclosporine is used to bring about a remission of psoriasis and maintenance therapy is continued with another treatment such as UVB or UVA and/or methotrexate or etretinate. In some cases, however, maintenance therapy may be continued with low dose Cyclosporine. Additionally, because each patient's dosage regimen may vary, you should discuss your exact course or therapy with your doctor.

As with all systemic treatments, Cyclosporine does have potential side effects. A temporary reduction in kidney function, which can be detected by laboratory tests, sometimes occurs with Cyclosporine. The drug has also been associated with permanent kidney damage. Kidney functions will be monitored by blood and urine tests throughout the treatment and Cyclosporine will be stopped if any significant changes occur.

Another risk is the development of lymphoma (cancer of the lymph glands) in patients who have received high doses of Cyclosporine, especially if they took other medications such as cortisone-like steroids. Therefore, you must not take any other immunosuppressants such as steroids while taking Cyclosporine. The doses of Cyclosporine you will be taking generally are lower than those given to transplant patients. It is not known if the risks of Cyclosporine causing lymphoma at these lower dosages are less. It is expected that they will be, but there is no current clinical proof. You will be monitored frequently to detect any signs of lymphoma.

Various forms of cancer (bladder, lung, breast and cervical cancer) have been observed in patients using Cyclosporine to treat psoriasis and other diseases.

Other potential side effects of Cyclosporine include: high blood pressure, increased hair growth, enlargement of the gums, headache, pain in the joints, tiredness, tingling in the fingers and toes, and shakiness. These side effects are usually associated with high doses of Cyclosporine and are reversible upon stopping or lowering the dose. Be sure to let your doctor know as soon as possible if you experience any of these side effects.

You must not take any nonsteroidal anti-inflammatory drugs such as aspirin, Advil or Motrin while taking Cyclosporine. Also you must not take medicines known to interact with Cyclosporine such as:

- Ketoconazole
- Erythromycin
- Phenytoin

- Barbiturates
- Carbamazepine
- Isoniazid
- Rifampicin

After the psoriasis has improved, patients are advised to switch to an alternate type of treatment. There are a number of other internal treatments for severe psoriasis. They include:

Azulfidine—occasionally useful for both arthritis and psoriasis. It can cause nausea and diarrhea, and some patients are allergic to it.

Hydroxyurea—an old-style anti-cancer drug which is sometimes mildly effective. Combining hydroxyurea with etretinate can boost its effectiveness. Blood counts should be monitored carefully while on this medication.

Azathioprine (also known as Immuran)—also an immune-suppressive drug, but not as powerful as Cyclosporine. Not as effective as etretinate, methotrexate or Cyclosporine. Azathioprine is occasionally used for patients with arthritis and severe skin psoriasis.

Dermatologists may sometimes prescribe other drugs such as the anti-cancer drug flourouracil, which can be used on a short-term basis. Cyclosporine is a very potent drug requiring frequent follow-up appointments and blood tests. Be sure to return to your doctor as scheduled. If you have any questions at any point during your treatment, be sure to ask your doctor.

SYSTEMIC STEROIDS

I have found that steroids taken internally to combat psoriasis have more pitfalls than benefits. (This is not true of topical steroids, which are very effective for many patients and which I discussed in Chapter 9.)

Too often, I have seen patients develop severe pustular and exfoliative reactions with their psoriasis when these systemic steroids have been discontinued. Some of the more common types of systemic steroids are prednisone (an oral medication), and triamcinolone (an intramuscular injection).

12

Future Hopes for Finding a Cure

While we do not yet know the cause of psoriasis, we do know much more today than we did a decade ago. Over the last ten years, scientists have discovered many of the skin changes now known to produce psoriasis. Among the most important recent discoveries are:

- Biochemical changes that may lead to the thickened skin and abnormal scale in psoriasis. This knowledge has led to new treatments that reduce this thickened skin and scale. It already has led to several new topical drugs that are being tested on patients. Some of these new treatments look very promising.
- Biochemical changes in the psoriasis skin that may cause or be part of the redness or inflammation. Understanding these has helped scientists develop new topical drugs (steroids and nonsteroidals) that have been made more effective in treating psoriasis. Some newer nonsteroidals may result in further improved treatments with fewer side effects for psoriasis skin.

· Immune changes that may produce the inflammation abnormalities mentioned above. Understanding these has already allowed an oral drug (Cyclosporine) to be extensively researched in patients with severe psoriasis.

These are exciting and hopeful times for medical research concerning psoriasis. New treatments are being discovered, existing treatments are being improved, future understanding about abnormalities in psoriasis will lead to new treatment approaches and hopefully control or clear the disease.

There are many new treatments for psoriasis. The following are just a few of the new therapies that are bringing hope to so many patients:

VITAMIN D ANALOGUES

Vitamin D analogues were also discussed in Chapter 9.

CALCIPOTRIOL OINTMENT

Recent research studies reported several types of Vitamin D-like drugs in both ointment and tablet form. One of these vitamin D-like drugs, called calcipotriol in the rest of the world and Calcipotriene ointment in the United States, is particularly exciting. The ointment works very well in about 70 percent of patients with plaque or patch type psoriasis. It has advantages over the cortisones because it does not cause skin thinning and this Vitamin D drug does not cause problems with any calcium buildup.

Recent research in Europe has determined that patients can use this ointment for long periods of time and that it significantly reduces the need for other treatments. Patients treating themselves with this ointment, in England, were able to drastically reduce the amount of the treatments and still keep control of their psoriasis. We expect that this ointment will be available in the United States sometime in 1993.

I have personally observed that calcipotriol ointment may be used effectively in combination with ultraviolet B (UVB) phototherapy and with psoralen in combination with ultraviolet A (PUVA) phototherapy.

Special Tips for Using calcipotriol/Calcipotriene (Dovonex) Ointment

- Small amounts of ointment should be applied only to the psoriasis plaques.
- Avoid putting it on the rest of the skin.
- Avoid putting any of the ointment in the skin folds, i.e., armpit and groin areas.
- Avoid putting the ointment on the face because it may cause some stinging and redness to the face.
- Use the ointment twice daily until the psoriasis is flattened and then reduce the frequency to once daily.
- You may sunbathe cautiously while you are using this ointment.
- If skin irritation or redness occurs see your dermatologist. Expect to see improvement with this ointment as early as one week. The maximum improvement may not be seen for about six to eight weeks.

TOPICAL RETINOIDS

Topical retinoids have been highly effective for a number of different skin diseases, including acne and ichthyoses, and in the treatment of photoaged skin. Several years ago, retinoic acid was also proven effective in treating psoriasis.

The main disadvantage of retinoic acid therapy in psoriasis is skin irritation. As a result, a search for retinoid analogues has resulted in agents that have retained a retinoid-like effect with less skin irritation. Recent controlled studies with a topical acetylenic retinoid have shown this agent to be effective in treating psoriasis.

Nonsteroidal Anti-Inflammatory Agents

We physicians continue to search for effective topical nonsteroidal anti-inflammatory agents to treat psoriasis. Nonsteroidal anti-inflammatory agents may have advantages over topical corticosteroids in that they are unlikely to cause skin atrophy. Newer agents under investigation show potential efficacy in psoriasis according to preliminary studies. One such drug that showed efficacy in Europe is Lonapalene.

NEW TRENDS IN THERAPY OF MORE SEVERE PSORIASIS

Recent trends in phototherapy have been designed to improve the efficacy of phototherapy and reduce toxicity. A drug called 8-MOP, dissolved in bathwater, is extremely valuable for patients who develop significant nausea from taking 8-MOP orally. Oral 5-methoxypsoralen (5-MOP) is as effective as 8-MOP PUVA, but appears to have a much lower risk of the acute toxicity problems of nausea.

There is hope that over the next few years we will make even greater strides toward curing psoriasis. Perhaps the most exciting research area for the future is the study of the gene or genes that, when inherited, may lead to psoriasis. The National Psoriasis Foundation in the U.S. has provided funds to help with this research, which will investigate families who have several members with psoriasis.

Recent research has shown that when animals have a gene added that is linked with a type of psoriasis arthritis, those animals develop the same disease that occurs in humans. Researchers have known for many years that psoriasis runs in families. More recent research has linked parts of chromosomes (the parts of the body cells that carry the genes) for psoriasis. Newer research techniques have made it possible to continue the search for abnormal or defective genes that are linked with psoriasis.

Time and more research are needed to isolate these abnormal genes. Once the abnormal gene or genes have been found, it will be necessary to determine how and why they do not work normally and what specific abnormality results. If this abnormality can be identified, researchers may be able to design treatments to correct it, and hopefully control psoriasis or even eradicate it.

13

Case Studies

Just as support groups may help you by allowing you to share with others who are going through the same things that you are, it can be helpful to know about psoriasis patients who have *already* gone through it and who successfully have come through treatment to feel better, more confident and more optimistic about controlling their disease in the long-run. The following actual case studies illustrate a range of psoriasis, from the localized but annoying disease to the more moderate but controllable cases, and finally to the more severe disabling type of psoriasis. You may well recognize details of your own disease. Psoriasis tends to follow several general patterns. Whether you recognize your own experiences in these or not, please recognize that today almost all forms of psoriasis can be controlled or cured completely. Thanks to new therapies and scientific knowledge, there is hope for every psoriasis patient.

CASE STUDY 1: LILLIAN

Lillian was 18 years old when she first developed psoriasis. It began four weeks after she had a severe but short-lived sore throat. Lillian had never seen psoriatic skin before (there was no family history of it) so she didn't know what was happening to her when she developed a large number of small, red, round scaling patches on her upper back. When the patches began spreading from her back to her thighs and arms, Lillian began to panic.

Initially, a family physician thought that Lillian's condition was a yeast infection of the skin, but when the scaling patches became thickened and more inflamed, he was baffled, and referred her to a dermatologist. The dermatologist diagnosed guttate psoriasis. This is the type of psoriasis that commonly follows a streptococcal sore throat and usually starts in childhood or during the teenage years.

Like many teenagers and young adults, Lillian was emotionally devastated by this outbreak of skin spots. She felt so unattractive and self-conscious that she had to take time off from work, and her boyfriend broke up with her. What had started as a few scaly patches was now a life-altering condition.

Lillian's dermatologist first treated her with a combination of oral antibiotics and intramuscular injections of a type of cortisone called kenalog. This improved her skin condition temporarily, but six weeks after the injection the skin spots returned even more severely.

That's when Lillian came to me for a new course of treatment. Because Lillian would have to take four weeks off from work to undergo my treatment plan, I wrote to her employer (with her permission), giving some details about her situation and explaining the need for her to attend my Treatment Center for coal tar ointment therapy.

Like other patients undergoing this therapy, Lillian came to the treatment center each day and stayed a minimum of three hours. When she arrived at the treatment center a nurse examined her and then applied special creams and ointments, each containing different concentrations of coal tar, over the entire surface of her affected skin. (These preparations are very messy, but can be used easily in a treatment center setting.) Lillian wore a special gown provided by the center to keep the cream and ointments in place. After two hours of being covered with the ointments Lillian showered and was then treated with carefully measured amounts of ultraviolet radiation in an ultraviolet cabinet. This combination-style treatment, known as the Goeckerman Treatment or Modified Goeckerman Therapy (after the dermatologist who devised it), has been used since the 1920s and is very effective.

Less than one month after beginning her daily treatments at the Center, Lillian's skin lesions were 90 percent cleared! At this point, she went back to work full-time. For another six weeks, Lillian came to the treatment center twice a week to receive an ultraviolet treatment lasting 10 minutes.

Since we stopped the treatments, Lillian has remained clear of any psoriasis. I explained to her that she may experience a recurrence, but if that happens, she knows to come to my office immediately to stop the disease from spreading. Lillian has also been given a supply of oral antibiotics to combat any threat of infection from future

87

sore throats. It is precisely this kind of infection that produced the severe type of guttate psoriasis she suffered.

CASE STUDY 2: BILL

Bill is a 35-year-old advertising executive who first developed psoriasis when he was 15. Fortunately, Bill's psoriasis
is confined to local scaling red patches on the elbows and
in the scalp. The patches on his scalp initially looked like
dandruff, with scale and flakes showing on Bill's dark business suits. He was able to control the scalp scaling with the
use of tar shampoos that he bought from the pharmacist.
However, his scalp became resistant to this shampoo
treatment over time, and the patches on his elbows began
to thicken.

Bill's main problem was the impact the scalp disease
had on his work. Although his colleagues never com-
mented on it, he knew they had all noticed his strange skin
disease. Some of them started shying away from him, and
he could see the questions in their eyes: Did he have a
fungus? Could he have AIDS?

As Bill became estranged from his co-workers, he lost a
lot of his confidence. He turned to his family practitioner,
who prescribed a variety of cortisone lotions for Bill to use
on the scalp twice a day. Unfortunately, many of these
lotions made his hair messy and greasy, and while they
worked initially, the scalp disease became resistant to their
effects.

Bill eventually heard about my treatment center from a
friend who also had psoriasis. After examining him, I offered Bill a choice of treatment options. We began by

trying local treatments to control his psoriasis. (I did not want to start him immediately on internal medications because of their side effects.) I selected a treatment using Anthralin—an old-fashioned treatment used since the late 1800s and by far the most common topical treatment for psoriasis in Europe.

Bill's elbow patches responded well to the Anthralin. But while that was a nice bonus, Bill's first priority was curing the scalp psoriasis. After nurses at the treatment center instructed Bill carefully in the use of the Anthralin scalp preparation, he began applying the liquid cream to his scalp every evening, keeping it on for increasing amounts of time, starting at 10 minutes and gradually working up to sessions of one hour or more. He shampooed the Anthralin off with tar shampoos containing salicylic acid. Over the next six weeks, Bill's scalp problem gradually improved, and he was able to reduce the frequency of the Anthralin scalp cream to once or twice a week.

Today, Bill still uses a tar shampoo every day. While it's likely that there will be times in the future when he will require more frequent treatments, Bill is greatly relieved by his progress to date. His relationships with colleagues have mended as well, so that the psoriasis no longer interferes with his work. Best of all, Bill has the secure knowledge that help is available should new outbreaks of his scalp disease occur.

CASE STUDY 3: PATRICK

Patrick was a healthy, slightly overweight 20-year-old with a family history of psoriasis. Both a brother and an uncle suffered from the disease. He developed psoriasis over most of his body after an initial patch appeared on his lower back, but he was able to cope with the familiar (and familial) disease until he developed a puzzling swelling and pain in his finger joints. This was the first sign that Patrick was developing arthritis as part of his psoriasis.

Only about 10 percent of psoriasis sufferers are afflicted by arthritis, but when psoriatic arthritis strikes, it can become very severe and disabling. Patrick became progressively immobilized by his dual diseases. His arthritis seemed to affect every joint, including his back. Because his knees and his shoulders were swollen and painful, his movement and activity level ground to a halt, and he was confined to bed for weeks at a time. Depressed and bored, Patrick ate to excess, put on weight, and was unable to continue with school or work because of his disabilities.

Patrick was referred to both a dermatologist and rheumatologist (arthritis expert). They initially treated him with arthritis medicine called Indocin, which had little impact on the arthritis, and may have even aggravated his skin problems. He was then treated with a drug called methotrexate which *did,* initially, help. Six months after treatment began, though, Patrick's doctors discovered that he had suffered liver damage as a result of the methotrexate and discontinued that therapy. At that point, Patrick almost despaired of receiving effective treatment.

But Patrick was referred to a psoriasis specialist who gave him Cyclosporine, which had shown great promise in Europe, and was then being investigated here in the U.S. Cyclosporine has been used since 1985 to combat the body's instinct to reject transplanted organs. Its application for psoriasis was discovered when two patients with psoriasis had organ transplants and were treated with it. Not only did Cyclosporine control the organ rejection, but it also dramatically improved their psoriasis.

Patrick took his Cyclosporine as a liquid dissolved in orange juice once in the morning and again in the evening. During the next three weeks his psoriasis markedly improved. He soon became more mobile, was able to walk again and even began attending physical therapy sessions to exercise.

Patrick continues to come to the office every four weeks so the staff can monitor his blood pressure, which up to now has been very well controlled. Once bedridden and despondent, Patrick is now optimistically considering his future career choices.

CASE STUDY 4: TED

Ted is a retired hardware-store owner. When he was 69, he developed scaling patches on his back and elbows, which his family physician correctly diagnosed as psoriasis. Initially, local cortisone creams and ointments controlled the condition. But then Ted's wife died, tragically and unexpectedly. He was devastated by his loss and began to drink heavily. About four months later, Ted's psoriasis began to spread and worsen.

A friend recommended one of the local psoriasis support groups of the National Psoriasis Foundation. (See the Appendix for further information on this foundation.) In turn, several members of the support group suggested that Ted see a psoriasis specialist.

By then, nearly 45 percent of Ted's skin was covered by the red scaling patches of psoriasis, many of them itchy and painful where they cracked. In discussing different treatment options, Ted said he really did not want to come into the hospital or spend long times at the treatment center. He still liked to go into his hardware store part-time and make sure everything was running smoothly.

Since Ted was clearly still emotionally distraught, the dermatologist suggested he see a psychiatrist in conjunction with his psoriasis treatment. The state of the skin and the psyche are frequently linked, and in Ted's case, it almost certainly was a combination of his wife's death and his psoriasis that caused his emotional distress.

Ted started a treatment program using PUVA (Psoralen-UVA phototherapy) at my treatment center and saw a counselor about his recent bereavement and the stress induced by his psoriasis. We hoped this plan would help Ted break the cycle of depression and psoriasis by attacking it from both sides.

Unfortunately, Ted became tired and nauseated about one hour after taking the psoralen pills that were required for his PUVA therapy (see Chapter 10 for further details on PUVA treatment). So at a follow-up visit, I instructed Ted to begin dissolving his medication in the bathwater instead of taking it in pill form; my research on PUVA treatment at that time suggested this might remedy these side effects.

Ted came to the treatment center three times a week for his 30-minute psoralen bath, followed immediately by 15 minutes in the UVA light. His psoriasis steadily improved on this regimen, and after six weeks I reduced his treatment to twice a week. Four weeks later, Ted was able to cut back to only one treatment a week.

Today, Ted maintains his weekly visits, which are sufficient to control his psoriasis. He may even be able to stop his PUVA therapy if he continues to improve. Many patients do remain clear after several months of the treatment. The psychological counseling has also proved beneficial. With more knowledge of his disease, Ted is better able to cope with the emotional disturbances psoriasis can cause and he has become more outgoing and socially involved.

CASE STUDY 5: SANDRA

Sandra was an 18–year–old high school student whose cousin had psoriasis. Sandra developed a sore throat that became very severe. Within two weeks of that sore throat she developed large numbers of flat, red, slightly scaly patches on the trunk and chest. Her family practitioner was unsure of the nature of the skin disease and she was referred to our dermatology center.

It was clear on taking her history and examining Sandra that she was suffering from a condition called guttate psoriasis. This frequently follows a "strep" or streptococcal sore throat.

We treated Sandra with the oral antibiotic erythromycin for her sore throat and with ultraviolet treatments three times per week. This resulted in significant improvement and clearance of her guttate psoriasis. Sandra has remained psoriasis-free for two years now. It is possible that she may get psoriasis in the future. In addition, if she gets any further sore throats she is to immediately start on her erythromycin antibiotic in an attempt to stop the occurrence of further guttate psoriasis.

CASE STUDY 6: STANLEY

Stanley was a 35–year–old who was referred to the dermatology center because of gradually worsening thick scaling patches on his elbows and scalp. His scalp scaling became so severe that his scalp felt as though it was enclosed in armor plated casing.

Because he had previously undergone multiple topical treatments for his scalp psoriasis, I decided to put Stanley on a low dosage of an oral medicine called etretinate. This is a Vitamin A-type derivative which can thin the thickened patches of scale in psoriasis. When the scale is thinned by this drug it can allow topical preparations such as the cortisone lotions and Anthralin scalp preparations to work much more efficiently.

Stanley still has his scalp psoriasis but it has improved sufficiently, and his outlook improved sufficiently. He is able to much more adequately cope with his disease.

CASE STUDY 7: PETER

Peter is a 20–year–old carpenter who developed scaling psoriasis patches on the knees and elbows. He also developed nail problems with his psoriasis and within six months started to develop arthritis in his fingers and toes. His psoriasis steadily worsened, despite topical treatment from his dermatologist. Peter was put on Indocin and other oral arthritis medicines. Unfortunately, his disease gradually worsened so that he was disabled from work because of his psoriasis of the nails, which became very painful, and because of the arthritis in his hands.

I decided, after careful history and discussion with Peter, that it was extremely important for him to be able to go back to work as soon as possible, and prescribed a drug called methotrexate, an anti-cancer drug that is used in psoriasis in very low dosages (usually between two and eight pills once to twice a week). It is very effective when there is plaque psoriasis and associated arthritis as in Peter's case.

Because methotrexate can affect the liver, I decided that it was necessary to see Peter every four weeks to repeat careful examination and to make sure that his blood tests were normal. It was also important to make sure that Peter did not drink alcohol or take any other medications for his psoriasis that might interfere with his methotrexate. These included large amounts of aspirins or other arthritis medication.

Peter is now back at work. He still has mild nail psoriasis but this has not been nearly as painful since starting his methotrexate. Peter is very pleased with his progress to date and I plan to keep him on methotrexate providing his blood tests stay normal and his liver biopsy is okay.

CASE STUDY 8: FRED

Fred is a 30–year–old research scientist who developed patches of psoriasis when he was a teenager. These became very persistent and always collected on the arms and legs. Although there were only about four patches, Fred was always embarrassed about them—especially around the women he was dating. Routine topical treatments such as topical cortisones did not clear Fred's patches, and Anthralin made the redness and inflammation much worse.

Serendipitously, Fred was planning to attend a scientific meeting in London. While there, I recommended that he see a friend and colleague of mine to obtain a prescription for calcipotriol (Dovonex) ointment. This Vitamin D analogue will, we hope, be available in the U.S. at the end of 1993. Unfortunately, it was not available in the U.S. when Fred needed it in 1992.

Calcipotriene ointment, as it will be known in the U.S., will enable patients to improve and control their psoriasis. It does not lead to skin thinning as with cortisone creams, nor does it stain the skin like coal tars or Anthralin. Fred was able to get this ointment from London and was allowed to bring it into this country for his own personal use. He has been applying it for two months and has already seen a very significant improvement in his psoriasis. We plan to continue this treatment on an as needed basis.

Questions and Answers About Psoriasis

Many of my patients have lots of questions about psoriasis. Here are some of the most common questions and their answers.

Q: Is psoriasis infectious or contagious?

A: Psoriasis is not infectious or contagious. You cannot infect others with it or contract it from other psoriasis sufferers. This is an important point that has to be reiterated frequently to family friends and employers who often worry needlessly. A dermatologist should be willing to provide a letter confirming this lack of infectiousness.

Q: Is psoriasis due to nerves, stress or other emotional factors?

A: Psoriasis is not caused by stress, but anxiety can and does aggravate the condition. Frequently several weeks or months pass after an especially stressful period before the psoriasis begins to worsen. Work-related stress, marital conflict and bereavement certainly can contribute to this problem. I once saw an example of this with a patient who had been under severe stress at work. His boss continually pressured him with unrealistic expectations and unfair deadlines. During a particularly pressure-filled period his psoriasis became much more severe with much larger areas of skin affected by psoriasis plaques. The patient left

97

his job to look for another one. His psoriasis grew even worse during this brief period of job hunting. Finally, when he settled into a new and more reasonable work environment, his psoriasis gradually improved and he needed fewer and fewer treatments.

Q: *Can diet improve my psoriasis?*

A: Many patients ask whether their unhealthful diets have caused their psoriasis or whether a particular diet can help their psoriasis. Diet is of course very important for the maintenance of good health, but it is unlikely to directly benefit psoriasis. However, it is known that diets containing high amounts of omega 3 polyunsaturated fats, such as fish oils, may help to reduce the inflammation caused not only by psoriasis but also by psoriatic arthritis. Omega 3 polyunsaturated fats are especially plentiful in salmon, herring, mackerel and other oily fish. (People who prefer to avoid these fatty fish could instead take fish oil capsules, which may produce the same effect.) A few of my patients have found that omitting pork from their diets has also helped.

Q: *I have a springtime allergy to grasses. My allergist suggested allergy-shot treatments until I told him that I had psoriasis. Can allergy-shot treatments aggravate my mild case of psoriasis?*

A: It is unlikely that injections that are intended to reduce your response to grass allergy will worsen your psoriasis. These injections generally are very small amounts of the allergic substance and are intended to produce a greater tolerance to the specific allergy. One of the treatments to avoid for severe allergies would be either intramuscular or systemic corticosteroid drugs e.g. prednisone or triamcinolone. These may temporarily improve your psoriasis, but subsequently your psoriasis may significantly worsen.

Q: *One day I decided to use the raw yoke of an egg on my psoriasis lesions. The itching stopped almost immediately and the scales are disappearing, so I have continued my egg treatments. What makes an egg yoke do this? Will there be any side effects?*

A: No one can say for sure what agent is likely to have produced the improvement in your psoriasis. Egg yolk contains large amounts of cholesterol and other lipids (fats). It is conceivable that the egg yolk was acting as a moisturizer and it is well known that moisturizers help to reduce the scale accumulation in psoriasis and other skin diseases. The most likely reason therefore is one of the effect of the lipid (fat) content of the egg yolk on your scales.

Q: *What side effects does methotrexate have on your liver?*

A: Methotrexate is a very effective drug for severe psoriasis and psoriatic arthritis. It can be used orally or by intramuscular or intralesional injections. It is very important for any doctor prescribing methotrexate to question you carefully about the possibility of liver disease. See Chapter 11 for more information about this drug.

Q: *I was diagnosed with psoriatic pubic symphysitis, an arthritis in the pelvic area that is extremely painful to me. Is there a particular treatment for this type of psoriatic*

99

arthritis? Is it common for psoriatic arthritis to occur in a man's pelvis?

A: Psoriatic arthritis can occur in any joint. While it is most common in the finger and toe joints, it can occur in the rib joints, between the ribs, and in the pubic area. The routine treatments for psoriatic arthritis in any area, include the use of a variety of nonsteroidal anti-inflammatory agents such as indomethacin, clinoral, voltarin, etc.

These drugs would be the first line of treatment. In patients with more severe and persistent arthritis, other agents that might be used include azulfidine, gold or methotrexate in low dosages. Seek the advice of both a dermatologist and a rheumatologist (joint arthritis expert) for your problem.

Q: My son is 12 years old and has had psoriasis since the age of four. My good news is that all of a sudden his psoriasis has improved 90 percent. He has not been on any oral medication except Naproxen for psoriatic arthritis and no topical cream except for moisturizing lotions. Could the varying hormone levels due to puberty have an effect on the psoriasis? My son hates to admit how improved his psoriasis is because he's afraid it will get worse again.

A: One of the great puzzles of psoriasis is what initiates spontaneous improvement in so many patients. It is very possible that a change in hormone pattern before puberty can influence psoriasis. We know, for example, that pregnant women often see changes in the severity of their psoriasis.

It is very understandable that your son is afraid that his

psoriasis will get worse again. Careful emotional support and reassurance should be given including the reassurance that there are numerous treatments that are available for psoriasis at the present time.

Q: What are Nystatin and Amphotericin B Cream? I have heard these mentioned as possible treatments for psoriasis and I was wondering if they could help me.

A: Nystatin is an agent that is effective against yeast infections including candida. Some researchers have suggested that there's a link between candida and psoriasis. These agents work in some patients particularly in the skin fold areas and the head areas such as the scalp.

Amphotericin B Cream, produced in France, is not the most effective treatment. I would recommend the Ketoconazole shampoo or broad spectrum imidazole creams (Spectazole, Oxystat, Nizoral, Micatin) instead.

Q: Do types of psoriasis change in an individual? For instance, if I have plaque psoriasis now, but sometimes it changes to guttate, and later on, to pustular. How common are these changes?

A: Some patients do have changing psoriasis during their lives and a number of different factors can change the pattern of psoriasis. For example streptococcal sore throats can produce a change of stable plaque psoriasis to guttate psoriasis. The excessive use of stronger topical corticosteroids for long periods or systemic steroids can occasionally produce changes to pustular psoriasis.

Certain medications such as lithium can change stable plaque psoriasis to pustular or severe exfoliative psoriasis. In many patients that have frequent changes to more severe pustular psoriasis, it is wise to try and treat the patients with anti–psoriasis treatments that will attempt to stabilize their disease. (Examples are if somebody is having recurrent pustular psoriasis to take low dosage systemic retinoids. If somebody is having recurrent guttate psoriasis then low dosage antibiotics such as erythromycin with frequent throat cultures and appropriate change to an alternative antibiotic are sometimes helpful.)

Q: Can skin that has been damaged by occlusive use of steroid creams be restored?

A: This depends on the degree of damage. Sometimes if the skin has been severely thinned by the steroids, it will not recover. But if the damage has been mild, stopping the corticosteroid or reducing the dosage to a much lower strength can help in skin recovery. There is additional research being conducted with agents such as topical retinoic acid in an attempt to see if that restores more rapidly the steroid induced skin thinning.

This is one of the reasons why great care needs to be taken with the use of topical steroids, particularly the strong ones used in the skin fold areas.

Q: Do animals get psoriasis, or is it only a human disease?

A: In fact there have been at least two reports of psoriasis or psoriasis–like conditions developing in rhesus monkeys. In addition, there are now genetically changed rats that have one of the genes added experimentally for psoriatic arthritis (the gene for HLA 27) that have been shown to develop a psoriasis–like condition. Further research in this area is extremely important and may lead to a greater understanding of the causes and the genetic control of psoriasis.

Q: *Why does my psoriasis get worse in the winter and better in the summer?*

A: We are not sure whether this common effect is a direct result of the amount of ultraviolet light available from the summer sun or whether it relates to the length of day. There are various theories about hormonal changes as well as a direct affect of ultraviolet light. While there is still a need for further research, the knowledge that psoriasis improves in the summer has led to the use of ultraviolet Phototherapy from artificial sunlamps in psoriasis. However, too much sunlight or artificial sunlight (ultraviolet) can lead to an increased risk of skin cancer, so it is important to consult your dermatologist for guidelines.

Q: *What factors can make my psoriasis worse?*

A: Several things are known to make psoriasis worse. These include medications including Beta blockers, lithium, antimalarial drugs as well as some anti-arthritis medications. A common factor in aggravating psoriasis, particularly in teenagers and younger adults, is streptococcal sore throats. These may result in a type of psoriasis called guttate (very small patches) of psoriasis. If you get strep throat, begin taking an antibiotic (either erythromycin or penicillin). Your physician can prescribe these for you and if you are highly susceptible to sore throats, you may want to keep some on hand at all times. Some physicians may not be aware of the link between strep and psoriasis, so it is important that you inform your doctor of your concerns about this.

Another thing that can produce psoriasis in about 30 percent of patients is skin damage. If you burn, cut or scrape the skin, psoriasis may occur in that part of damaged skin. This is known as Koebner's phenomenon. It is very important for anybody with psoriasis to carefully avoid skin damage, for example, abrasions, burns etc.

Nail psoriasis can also be made worse by a Koebner–type reaction, so do not scrape or clean under the nails or damage the nail in any way. If you are going to be working in the yard or at a manual job, use gloves to protect the nails as much as possible and reduce the risk of further nail damage with psoriasis.

Q: *What do the terms "steroids" and "cortisones" mean? Are these dangerous for psoriasis patients?*

A: Cortisones and steroids are common names for treatments used for a variety of diseases. Cortisones are mainly used for the treatment of inflammatory diseases. The steroids or cortisones that are used for skin diseases are not related to the anabolic cortisones or anabolic steroids that are used (and misused) by some athletes for muscle building.

Psoriasis patients should avoid systemic (intramuscular or oral) cortisones wherever possible. (There are a few exceptions such as patients with severe arthritis or other diseases such as severe asthma that may occasionally need these drugs.) These drugs may drastically worsen the psoriasis in ways that we do not understand. After taking these internal or systemic cortisones, the psoriasis can become extremely severe and unstable.

Topical cortisones in creams, ointments and lotions are

extremely helpful for many patients with psoriasis. However, even these need to be carefully used to avoid side effects. Side effects include excessive thinning of the skin (particularly in the skin folds and face area), and excessive appearance of blood vessels where the skin is thinned. This is very noticeable at times on the face. In addition, skin infections and hair follicle infections can produce problems with excessive topical cortisone use. Talk to your dermatologist about which cortisone you should use, and how. Generally, you will use the mildest cortisones i.e., one-percent hydrocortisone cream or ointment on the face, skin folds and genital area. Stronger cortisones will generally be needed on other parts of the body.

Q: I have psoriatic arthritis. Will my arthritis get worse with my psoriasis?

A: Psoriatic arthritis generally does get worse following worsening psoriasis. There are a few patients who have psoriatic arthritis without any evidence of skin psoriasis. In general, however, they will develop skin psoriasis at some stage. Remember to protect the joints as much as possible when you have acute arthritis.

Q: Will my psoriasis get worse if I am pregnant?

A: Many psoriatic women who become pregnant do experience changes in their psoriasis. The psoriasis usually improves considerably during pregnancy. Unfortunately, it will frequently get worse in the months following delivery. If you are pregnant or likely to become pregnant, DO NOT use medications that can potentially harm the developing child. These medications include any of the internal medications such as methotrexate, Retinoids and Cyclosporine. Additionally, it is probably unwise to receive PUVA phototherapy or apply excessive amounts of topical medications. Fertile and pregnant women can usually use small amounts of topical corticosteroids, small quantities of Anthralin cream or ointment and as much moisturizer as they desire. Speak to your obstetrician about any medications you are using.

Q: *How common is psoriasis?*

A: Psoriasis is a very common disease affecting approximately two percent of the population. This means that one in 50 people has psoriasis or approximately five to six million people in the U.S.

It is often helpful for people with psoriasis to realize that there are many others with the disease in the community.

Q: *Should I wash with soap if I have psoriasis?*

A: It is best to use relatively mild soaps for any skin disease. Non-detergent soap substitutes may be less drying and less irritating. Examples of these soap substitutes are Cetaphil or Aquanil.

In addition, soaps or bath oils that contain coal tars or moisturizers such as Balnetar or Polytar are very helpful as agents to soothe skin within psoriasis.

Appendix

USEFUL ADDRESSES OF PSORIASIS ASSOCIATIONS FOR THE
PSORIASIS PATIENT WORLDWIDE

United States
The National Psoriasis
  Foundation
6600 SW 92nd Ave.
Suite 300
Portland, OR 97223

Australia
The Skin and Psoriasis
  Foundation
P.O. Box 228
PO Collins Street
3000 Melbourne

Belgium
Vlaamse Vereniging Psoriasis
  Patineten
Heedstraat 33—1730 Asse

GIPSO
30 rue de l'Armistice
4020 Liege

Canada
Canadian Psoriasis Foundation
1565 Carling Avenue
Suite 400
Ottawa
Ontario, K1Z 8R1

The Canadian Psoriasis
  Association
The Women's College Hospital
76 Greenville Street
Toronto, Ontario

Psoriasis Society of Canada
P.O. Box 9551
Station A
Halifax, Nova Scotia B3K 5S4

Croatia
Dristvo Psorijaticara I Irvatske
Svarcova ul. 20
41000 Zagreb

Czechoslovakia
The Society of Psoriasis in
  Czechozlovakie
Struharovska 2941
14100 Prague

Denmark
Danmarks Psoriasis Forening
Landskronagade 66.4
2100 Kobenhavno

Egypt
Egyptian Psoriasis Society
P.O. Box 29
Citadel
Cairo

Estonia
Eesti Psoriaasi Lut
Kulmaallika 8A
200026 Tallinn

Finland
The Finnish Psoriasis
    Association
Fredrikinkatu 27 A 1,
00120 Helsinki

France
Association Pour La Lutte
    Contre Le Psoriasis
1 Rue des Bois
95520 OSNY

Germany
Duetscher Psoriasis Bund E.V.
Oberaltenallee 20A
2000 Hamburg 76

PSO Aktuell
Postfach 43 06 29
D-8000 Munchen 43

Great Britain
The Psoriasis Association
7 Milton Street
Northampton NN2 75G

Iceland
Samtok Psoriasis
Og Exemsjuklinga (Spoex)
Bolholt 6, 105 Reykjavik

Israel
Israel Psoriasis Association
P.O. Box 13275
Tel-Aviv

Italy
ASN
Via Bergogne 43
20114 Milano

ADIPSO
Via Cavour 266
00134 Roma
APSIAR
Clinica dermatologica dell
    Universita—34100
Trieste

Jordan
Jordanian Psoriasis
    Association
P.O. Box 184 194
Amman

Netherlands
Nederlandse Bond van
    Psoriasis
Patientenverenigingen (NBPV)
Bouriciussur 4—6014 CW
ARWNHEM

New Zealand
The Auckland Psoriasis
    Society
P.O. Box 3062
Auckland I

Norway
Norsk Psoriasis Forbund
Grenseveien 86 A
0663 Oslo

Portugal
Associacao Dos Psoriaticos de
   Portugal
1 Esq. Rhua Almeida
Garrette 47
8000 Faro

Singapore
Psoriasis Association of
   Singapore
National Skin Center
C/O Phototherapy Unit
No. 1 Mandalay Road
1130

South Africa
The South African Psoriasis
   Association
106 H Baker Street
Groenkloof
Pretoria 0181

Sweden
Svenska Psoriasisforbundet
Sveavagen 31
111 34 Stockholm

Switzerland
Schweizerische Psoriasis-
   Gesellschaft
Postfach 8027
Zurich

Venezuela
Venezuela National Psoriasis
   Foundation
Centro Clinico Professional
AV. Phanteon,
San Bernardino
Piso 3, Consultoio 304
Caracas

ADDITIONAL SOURCES OF INFORMATION IN THE U.S.

The National Psoriasis Foundation is located at 6600 S.W. 92nd Avenue, Suite 300, Portland, OR 97223. As a NPF member, you can receive numerous booklets dealing with psoriasis and related issues. For the cost of annual membership, which is a donation of any amount, members receive *Bulletin,* a newsletter that offers news on current treatments and research; educational literature— numerous booklets on a wide range of specific topics; *Pharmacy News,* a newsletter that announces new or unique products, lists over-the-counter and prescription psoriasis medications and also contains interesting articles. This publication is sent to members three times a year. These are just a sample of the items and services available from the NPF. The NPF can be reached by calling (503) 244-7404.

The American Academy of Dermatology. The AAD has a consumer pamphlet on psoriasis that is available by sending a self-addressed, stamped, business-size envelope to: AAD, P.O. Box 4014, Schaumburg, IL 60168-4014. Mark it "Psoriasis." The AAD also offers nearly 40 consumer pamphlets on a variety of skin and hair disorders.

The Skin Research Foundation of California is dedicated to supporting research on a number of skin diseases. The foundation supports physician and public education about psoriasis and other diseases, including sponsorship of psoriasis support groups. For further information call (310) 828-8969.

Index

About the Author

Dr. Nicholas J. Lowe, M.D., is a dermatologist in private practice in Santa Monica and Westlake, CA. He also is medical director of the Skin Research Foundation of California, which is dedicated to research and education of skin diseases. He is also Clinical Professor of Dermatology at the UCLA School of Medicine, Los Angeles, CA.

Dr. Lowe has for 20 years been involved in dermatology as a researcher, teacher and physician treating patients. He first became interested in dermatology after training as a specialist in internal medicine in Great Britain, where he established one of the first phototherapy units in that country. He also has helped to develop and improve treatment for psoriasis called PUVA phototherapy which involves the activation of medication by ultraviolet radiation in the skin. One of the great advantages of phototherapy is that it is capable of treating the whole skin and does not lead to any known internal complications.

Dr. Lowe received a research fellowship in 1975 at Scripps Clinic and Research Foundation and the University of California, San Diego in La Jolla. This fellowship sparked a continuing interest in new treatments for psoriasis and the best way of critically studying them.

For more than 10 years he was professor of dermatology at the UCLA School of Medicine, where he established both a research program in psoriasis therapy as well as the medical school's first comprehensive psoriasis treatment center.

In 1988 he founded the Southern California Dermatology and Psoriasis Centers in Santa Monica and Westlake, based on his many years of experience in treating this disease in both Britain and the United States. The Centers offer a wide variety of psoriasis treatments and are two of very few in Southern California with day therapy facilities.

Additional copies of *Managing Your Psoriasis* may be ordered by sending a check for $10.95 (please add the following for postage and handling: $2.00 for the first copy, $1.00 for each added copy) to:

MasterMedia Limited
17 East 89th Street
New York, NY 10128
(212) 260-5600
(800) 334-8232
fax: (212) 546-7638

The author is available for workshops, seminars, and speeches. Please contact MasterMedia's Speakers' Bureau for availability and fee arrangements. Call Tony Colao at (800) 4-LECTUR; fax: (908) 359-1647.

Other MasterMedia Books

To order MasterMedia books, either go to your local bookstore or call (800) 334-8232.

THE PREGNANCY AND MOTHERHOOD DIARY: Planning the First Year of Your Second Career, by Susan Schiffer Stautberg, is the first and only undated appointment diary that shows how to manage pregnancy and career. ($12.95 spiral-bound)

CITIES OF OPPORTUNITY: Finding the Best Place to Work, Live and Prosper in the 1990's and Beyond, by Dr. John Tepper Marlin, explores the job and living options for the next decade and into the next century. This consumer guide and handbook, written by one of the world's experts on cities, selects and features forty-six American cities and metropolitan areas. ($13.95 paper, $24.95 cloth)

THE DOLLARS AND SENSE OF DIVORCE, by Dr. Judith Briles, is the first book to combine practical tips on overcoming the legal hurdles by planning finances before, during, and after divorce. ($10.95 paper)

OUT THE ORGANIZATION: New Career Opportunities for the 1990's, by Robert and Madeleine Swain, is written for the millions of Americans whose jobs are no longer safe, whose companies are not loyal, and who face futures of uncertainty. It gives advice on finding a new job or starting your own business. ($12.95 paper)

AGING PARENTS AND YOU: A Complete Handbook to Help You Help Your Elders Maintain a Healthy, Productive and Independent Life, by Eugenia Anderson-Ellis, is a complete guide to providing care to aging relatives. It gives practical advice and resources to the adults who are helping their elders lead productive and independent lives. Revised and updated. ($9.95 paper)

CRITICISM IN YOUR LIFE: How to Give It, How to Take It, How to Make It Work for You, by Dr. Deborah Bright, offers practical advice, in an upbeat, readable, and realistic fashion, for turning criticism into control. Charts and diagrams guide the reader into managing criticism from bosses, spouses, children, friends, neighbors, in-laws, and business relations. ($17.95 cloth)

BEYOND SUCCESS: How Volunteer Service Can Help You Begin Making a Life Instead of Just a Living, by John F. Raynolds III and Eleanor Raynolds, C.B.E., is a unique how-to book targeted at business and professional people considering volunteer work, senior citizens who wish to fill leisure time meaningfully, and students trying out various career options. The book is filled with interviews with celebrities, CEOs, and average citizens who talk about the benefits of service work. ($19.95 cloth)

MANAGING IT ALL: Time-Saving Ideas for Career, Family, Relationships, and Self, by Beverly Benz Treuille and Susan Schiffer Stautberg, is written for women who are juggling careers and families. Over two hundred career women (ranging from a TV anchorwoman to an investment banker) were interviewed. The book contains many humorous anecdotes on saving time and improving the quality of life for self and family. ($9.95 paper)

YOUR HEALTHY BODY, YOUR HEALTHY LIFE: How to Take Control of Your Medical Destiny, by Donald B. Louria, M.D., provides precise advice and strategies that will help you to live a long and healthy life. Learn also about nutrition, exercise, vitamins, and medication, as well as how to control risk factors for major diseases. Revised and updated. ($12.95 paper)

THE CONFIDENCE FACTOR: How Self-Esteem Can Change Your Life, by Dr. Judith Briles, is based on a nationwide survey of six thousand men and women. Briles explores why women so often feel a lack of self-confidence and have a poor opinion of themselves. She offers step-by-step advice on becoming the person you want to be. ($9.95 paper, $18.95 cloth)

THE SOLUTION TO POLLUTION: 101 Things You Can Do to Clean Up Your Environment, by Laurence Sombke, offers step-by-step techniques on how to conserve more energy, start a recycling center, choose biodegradable products, and even proceed with individual environmental cleanup projects. ($7.95 paper)

TAKING CONTROL OF YOUR LIFE: The Secrets of Successful Enterprising Women, by Gail Blanke and Kathleen Walas, is based on the authors' professional experience with Avon Products' Women of Enterprise Awards, given each year to outstanding women entrepreneurs. The authors offer a specific plan to help you gain control over your life, and include business tips and quizzes as well as beauty and lifestyle information. ($17.95 cloth)

SIDE-BY-SIDE STRATEGIES: How Two-Career Couples Can Thrive in the Nineties, by Jane Hershey Cuozzo and S. Diane Graham, describes how two-career couples can learn the difference between competing with a spouse and becoming a supportive power partner. Published in hardcover as *Power Partners.* ($10.95 paper, $19.95 cloth)

DARE TO CONFRONT! How to Intervene When Someone You Care About Has an Alcohol or Drug Problem, by Bob Wright and Deborah George Wright, shows the reader how to use the step-by-step methods of professional interventionists to motivate drug-dependent people to accept the help they need. ($17.95 cloth)

WORK WITH ME! How to Make the Most of Office Support Staff, by Betsy Lazary, shows you how to find, train, and nurture the "perfect" assistant and how to best utilize your support staff professionals. ($9.95 paper)

MANN FOR ALL SEASONS: Wit and Wisdom from The Washington Post's *Judy Mann,* by Judy Mann, shows the columnist at her best as she writes about women, families, and the impact and politics of the women's revolution. ($9.95 paper, $19.95 cloth)

THE SOLUTION TO POLLUTION IN THE WORKPLACE, by Laurence Sombke, Terry M. Robertson and Elliot M. Kaplan, supplies employees with everything they need to know about cleaning up their workspace, including recycling, using energy efficiently, conserving water and buying recycled products and nontoxic supplies. ($9.95 paper)

THE ENVIRONMENTAL GARDENER: The Solution to Pollution for Lawns and Gardens, by Laurence Sombke, focuses on what each of us can do to protect our endangered plant life. A practical sourcebook and shopping guide. ($8.95 paper)

THE LOYALTY FACTOR: Building Trust in Today's Workplace, by Carol Kinsey Goman, Ph.D., offers techniques for restoring commitment and loyalty in the workplace. ($9.95 paper)

DARE TO CHANGE YOUR JOB—AND YOUR LIFE, by Carole Kanchier, Ph.D., provides a look at career growth and development throughout the life cycle. ($9.95 paper)

MISS AMERICA: In Pursuit of the Crown, by Ann-Marie Bivans, is an authorized guidebook to the Pageant, containing eyewitness accounts, complete historical data, and a realistic look at the trials and triumphs of the potential Miss Americas. ($19.95 paper, $27.50 cloth; b&w and color photos)

POSITIVELY OUTRAGEOUS SERVICE: New and Easy Ways to Win Customers for Life, by T. Scott Gross, identifies what the consumers of the nineties really want and how businesses can develop effective marketing strategies to answer those needs. ($14.95 paper)

BREATHING SPACE: Living and Working at a Comfortable Pace in a Sped-Up Society, by Jeff Davidson, helps readers to handle information and activity overload, and gain greater control over their lives. ($10.95 paper)

TWENTYSOMETHING: Managing and Motivating Today's New Work Force, by Lawrence J. Bradford, Ph.D., and Claire Raines, M.A., examines the work orientation of the younger generation, offering managers in businesses of all kinds a practical guide to better understand and supervise their young employees. ($22.95 cloth)

REAL LIFE 101: The Graduate's Guide to Survival, by Susan Kleinman, supplies welcome advice to those facing "real life" for the first time, focusing on work, money, health, and how to deal with freedom and responsibility. ($9.95 paper)

BALANCING ACTS! Juggling Love, Work, Family, and Recreation, by Susan Schiffer Stautberg and Marcia L. Worthing, provides strategies to achieve a balanced life by reordering priorities and setting realistic goals. ($12.95 paper)

REAL BEAUTY . . . REAL WOMEN: A Handbook for Making the Best of Your Own Good Looks, by Kathleen Walas, International Beauty and Fashion Director of Avon Products, offers expert advice on beauty and fashion to women of all ages and ethnic backgrounds. ($19.50 paper; in full color)

THE LIVING HEART BRAND NAME SHOPPER'S GUIDE (Revised and Updated), by Michael E. DeBakey, M.D., Antonio M. Gotto, Jr., M.D., D.Phil., Lynne W. Scott, M.A., R.D./L.D., and John P. Foreyt, Ph.D., lists brand-name supermarket products that are low in fat, saturated fatty acids, and cholesterol. ($14.95 paper)

MANAGING YOUR CHILD'S DIABETES, by Robert Wood Johnson IV, Sale Johnson, Casey Johnson, and Susan Kleinman, brings help to families trying to understand diabetes and control its effects. ($10.95 paper)

STEP FORWARD: Sexual Harassment in the Workplace, What You Need to Know, by Susan L. Webb, presents the facts for identifying the tell-tale signs of sexual harassment on the job, and how to deal with it. ($9.95 paper)

A TEEN'S GUIDE TO BUSINESS: The Secrets to a Successful Enterprise, by Linda Menzies, Oren S. Jenkins, and Rickell R. Fisher, provides solid information about starting a business or working for one. ($7.95 paper)

GLORIOUS ROOTS: Recipes for Healthy, Tasty Vegetables, by Laurence Sombke, celebrates the taste, texture, and versatility of root vegetables. Contains recipes for appetizers, soups, stews, and baked, boiled, and stir-fried dishes—even desserts. ($12.95 paper)

THE OUTDOOR WOMAN: A Handbook to Adventure, by Patricia Hubbard and Stan Wass, details the lives of adventurous outdoor women and offers their ideas on how you can incorporate exciting outdoor experiences into your life. ($14.95 paper; with photos)

FLIGHT PLAN FOR LIVING: The Art of Self-Encouragement, by Patrick O'Dooley, is a life-guide organized like a pilot's flight checklist, which ensures you'll be flying "clear on top" throughout your life. ($17.95 cloth)

HOW TO GET WHAT YOU WANT FROM ALMOST ANYBODY, by T. Scott Gross, shows how to get great service, negotiate better prices, and always get what you pay for. ($9.95 paper)

TEAMBUILT: Making Teamwork Work, by Mark Sanborn, teaches business how to improve productivity, without increasing resources or expenses, by building teamwork among employers. ($19.95 cloth)

THE BIG APPLE BUSINESS AND PLEASURE GUIDE: 501 Ways to Work Smarter, Play Harder, and Live Better in New York City, by Muriel Siebert and Susan Kleinman, offers visitors and New Yorkers alike advice on how to do business in the city as well as how to enjoy its attractions. ($9.95 paper)

FINANCIAL SAVVY FOR WOMEN: A Money Book for Women of All Ages, by Dr. Judith Briles, provides a critical and in-depth look at financial structures and tools any woman wanting to achieve total independence can use. ($14.95 paper)

MIND YOUR OWN BUSINESS: And Keep It in the Family, by Marcy Syms, COO of Syms Corporation, is an effective guide for any organization, small or large, facing what is documented to be the toughest step in managing a family business—making the transition to the new generation. ($18.95 cloth)

KIDS WHO MAKE A DIFFERENCE, by Joyce M. Roché and Marie Rodriguez with Phyllis Schneider, is a surprising and inspiring document of some of today's toughest challenges being met—by teen-agers and kids! Their courage and creativity allowed them to find practical solutions. ($8.95 paper; with photos)

ROSEY GRIER'S ALL-AMERICAN HEROS: Multicultural Success Stories, by Roosevelt "Rosey" Grier, is a wonderful collection of personal histories, told in their own words, by prominent African-Americans, Latins, Asians, and Native Americans; all tell of the people in their lives and choices they made in achieving public acclaim and personal success. ($9.95 paper; with portrait photos)

OFFICE BIOLOGY: Why Tuesday Is the Most Productive Day and Other Relevant Facts for Survival in the Workplace, by Edith Weiner and Arnold Brown, teaches how in the '90s and beyond we will be expected to work smarter, take better control of our health, adapt to advancing technology, and improve our lives in ways that are not too costly or resource-intensive. ($21.95 cloth)

ON TARGET: Enhance Your Life and Ensure Your Success, by Jeri Sedlar and Rick Miners, is a neatly woven tapestry of insights on career and life issues gathered from audiences across the country. This feedback has been crystalized into a highly readable guidebook for exploring who you are and how to go about getting what you want from your career and your life. ($11.95 paper)

SOMEONE ELSE'S SON, by Alan A. Winter, explores the parent-child bond in a contemporary story of lost identities, family secrets, and relationships gone awry. Eighteen years after bringing their first son home from the hospital, Trish and Brad Hunter discover they are not his natural parents. Torn between their love for their son, Phillip, and the question of whether they should help him search for his biological parents, the couple must also struggle with the issue of their own biological son. Who is he—and do his parents know their baby was switched at birth? ($18.95 cloth)

STRAIGHT TALK ON WOMEN'S HEALTH: How to Get the Health Care You Deserve, by Janice Teal, Ph.D., and Phyllis Schneider, is destined to become a health-care "bible" for women concerned about their bodies and their future health. Well-researched, but devoid of confusing medical jargon, this handbook offers access to a wealth of resources, with a bibliography of health-related books and contact lists of organizations, healthlines, and women's medical centers. ($14.95 paper)

THE STEPPARENT CHALLENGE: A Primer for Making It Work, by Stephen J. Williams, Sc.D., shares firsthand experience and insights into the many aspects of dealing with step relationships—from financial issues to lifestyle changes to differences in race or religion that affect the whole family. Peppered with personal accounts and useful tips, this volume is must reading for anyone who is a stepparent, about to become one, or planning to bring children to a second or subsequent marriage. ($13.95 paper)

PAIN RELIEF! How to Say No to Acute, Chronic, and Cancer Pain, by Dr. Jane Cowles, offers a step-by-step plan for assessing pain and communicating it to your doctor, and explains the importance of having a pain plan before undergoing any medical or surgical treatment. This landmark book includes "The Pain Patient's Bill of Rights," and a reusable pain assessment chart designed to help patients and their families make informed decisions. ($22.95 cloth)

MAKING YOUR DREAMS COME TRUE: A Plan for Easily Discovering and Achieving the Life You Want, by Marcia Wieder, introduces an easy, unique, and practical technique for defining, pursuing, and realizing your career and life interests. Filled with stories of real people and helpful exercises, plus a personal workbook, this clever volume will teach you how to make your dreams come true—any time you choose. ($9.95 paper)

WHAT KIDS LIKE TO DO, by Edward Stautberg, Gail Wubbenhorst, Atiya Easterling, and Phyllis Schneider, is a handy guidebook for parents, grandparents, and babysitters who are searching for activities that kids *really* enjoy. Written by kids for kids, this easy-to-read, generously illustrated primer can teach families how to make every day more fun. ($7.95 paper)

THE LIVING HEART GUIDE TO EATING OUT, by Michael E. De-Bakey, M.D., Antonio M. Gotto, Jr., M.D., D.Phil., and Lynne W. Scott, M.A., R.D./L.D., is the first complete guide to heart-healthy foods in ethnic restaurants (Chinese, Italian, Mexican, etc.) and when traveling (airline meals). ($9.95 purse-size paperback; available October 1993)